BESTFEEDING:
Getting Breastfeeding Right for You

The Illustrated Guide

By Mary Renfrew
Chloe Fisher and Suzanne Arms

CELESTIALARTS
Berkeley, California

CELESTIALARTS

P.O. Box 7123
Berkeley, California 94707
United States of America

Cover photo by SuperStock
Cover and text design by Brad Greene
Composition by Greene Design

Library of Congress Cataloging-in-Publication Data

Renfrew, Mary, 1955–
        Bestfeeding : getting breastfeeding right for you : an illustrated
guide / by Mary Renfrew, Chloe Fisher, and Suzanne Arms.
            p. cm.
        Previously published: 1990.
        Includes bibliographical references and index.
        ISBN 0-89087-955-9 (pbk.)
        1. Breast feeding—Popular works. I. Fisher, Chloe, 1932– II. Arms,
Suzanne. III. Title.

RJ216 .R385 2000
649'.33—dc21   00-035822

    2 3 4 5 6 — 02 01 00
Manufactured in the United States of America

This book is dedicated
to all women
who have had problems with breastfeeding—
to those who struggled on despite difficulties,
and to those who gave up breastfeeding
before they wanted to

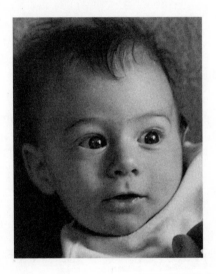

It is also dedicated with affection
and respect
to
Dr. Mavis Gunther,
whose work started us on the right road.

Contents

CHAPTER 4

CHAPTER 5

CHAPTER 6

CHAPTER 7

CHAPTER 8

CHAPTER 9
THE TEN BASIC STEPS: A STORYBOARD

Acknowledgments

Like breastfeeding itself, this book needed support, and it benefited from the wisdom and guidance of skilled helpers. We were privileged to have the help of many people throughout the world in its preparation. The information we offer is based on clinical and personal experience, as well as a great deal of research. We are especially indebted to the work of Kathy Auerbach, Maureen Minchin and Mike Woolridge, whose understanding of breastfeeding and creativity in the field has contributed much to this book.

Most of what we have learned about breastfeeding has come from mothers, from fathers, and from babies. We want to acknowledge all the families we have worked with through the years. Our special thanks go to the women and families who allowed us to photograph them for this book: Sparrow Baranyai and Gary Blackburn, Martha Lopez-Chubb, Jackie and Larry Foreman, Christine Hunner, Judith Landy, Jenchyn and Raymond Luh, Lorri and Diego Roa, Lawan Jackson, Ann Marie Joyce, and Lesley Searle.

Many people read and commented on the text, and in so doing made it better. For correcting our errors, challenging our assumptions, and helping keep dogma to a minimum, we sincerely thank Kathy Auerbach, David Baum, Maggie Conroy, Donna Cowan, Susan Currie, Jo Garcia, Faye Gibson, Lynne Gleason, Karyn Kaufman, Brian McClelland, Kathy Michaelson, Maureen Minchin, Jane Morton, Gay Palmer, Harriet Palmer, and Mike Wooldridge. Thank you, Barbara Henry and Shirley Anne Seel, for help with the resources section.

Special thanks to Maria Tiscareno for the Spanish translation of concepts in the storyboard.

Our publishers believed in us and supported us all along the way in our efforts to create an inexpensive yet lavishly beautiful book. Thank you, David Hinds and Paul Reed of Celestial Arts. Thank you also to The Department of Health, England, which supported Mary Renfrew during the writing of this book, and to everyone at the National Perinatal Epidemiology Unit at Oxford for their understanding and practical support.

We have had lots of personal support as well, from our family and friends. All of them believed in and encouraged us, even when our work on this book got in the way of time they wanted to spend with us. A special thanks, John Wimberley, for allowing us to take over your home while we wrote, held meetings, and conducted interviews with breastfeeding mothers. Thanks for cups of tea and hugs, for making us laugh, and for giving us the brilliant title for this book.

Our own mothers were all strong women who wanted to breastfeed their babies but lived during times when breastfeeding was difficult. We are grateful for their perseverance in trying to do what was best for their children, and for their strong influence on our lives.

Some places too have been special to us in the creation of this book. Without a visit to Glastonbury, England, the book might never have been conceived. We worked together in Oxford, England, and in Palo Alto, California, and both of these places influenced our work, giving us the pleasure of long walks and magnificent skies.

More than anything, the joy of this book for us has been our collaboration with each other. Our different backgrounds, experiences, and ages have made our work together special, and we have learned a great deal from each other. For all of this we are most grateful.

Acknowledgments for Second Edition

Revising this book to produce the second edition has been an ongoing process over several years. Many of the women who have read this book have contributed to that process, by taking the time to write to us to tell us about what was important to them, and to give us their suggestions for making the book better.

Many of the changes in the book reflect the changes in our own lives over the years. Mary has had two children, Jamie and Calum, who have taught her more about birth, breastfeeding and parenting than anyone else ever could. They also brought Chloe some new challenges—she supported Mary with her breastfeeding—as they presented some new situations which Chloe had not encountered before. Thank you, boys, for bringing us joy, making us question what we thought we knew, and never letting us become complacent.

Chloe has retired, but continues to work with women almost every day. Thanks to the John Radcliffe Hospital in Oxford, England, where Chloe still runs her breastfeeding clinic, along with her colleague, Sally Inch.

Suzanne has moved to live in Colorado, where she works closely with her husband, Root Routledge. Thanks to him and to the staff with whom they work, for their love and support.

Several people have helped in the practical process of producing this new book. Phil Minchin helped to update the resource section. Helen Bridges worked tirelessly on the manuscript. Mary's colleagues at the Mother and Infant Research Unit in the University of Leeds were a constant source of support, and the University of Leeds supported her while she was working on this new edition.

Our colleagues and friends commented on the changes in the book. For correcting out errors and making it a better book, thanks to Jim Akre, Caroline Harris, and Randa Saadeh. Any remaining errors are, of course, our responsibility.

We have had support and practical help from our publishers, Celestial Arts. Thanks especially to Veronica Randall for keeping us (almost) to schedule.

Our work over these years has been especially challenging as we have not had the opportunity to all be together at the same time. We have worked by telephone, fax and email—a surprisingly easy process. We are grateful to the new technologies for assisting us, and we have included references to Internet resources in the book for those with access to them.

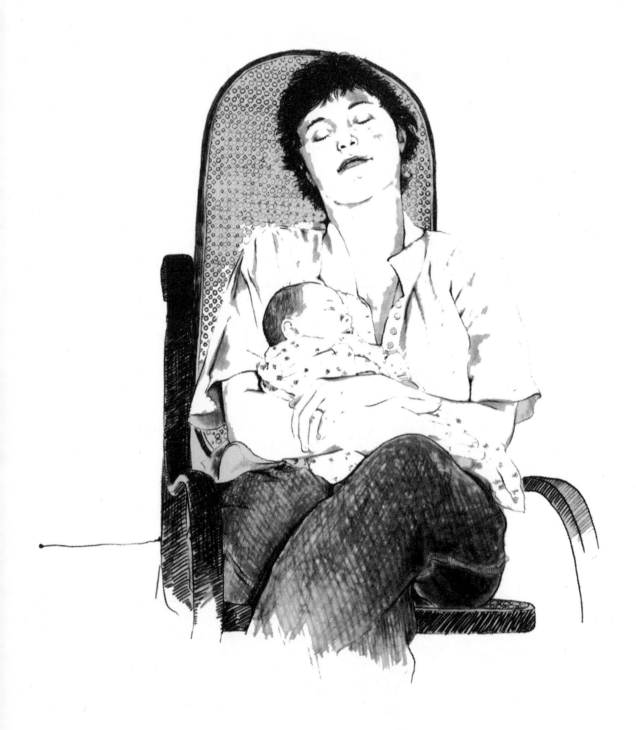

About This Book

What This Book Contains

Breastfeeding is by far the best way to feed a baby. Many women know this. But breastfeeding is not always easy for women who live in societies where it is hidden, and we don't get a chance to learn how to do it. Some women find that breastfeeding is easy and satisfying, right from the start. But many women in industrialized countries find it difficult to do without help. And it can be hard to find the right help. It is important to understand that knowing how to breastfeed is not something you are born with; it is something you learn. On the other hand babies are born knowing how to do their part; but they need your help.

This book is about getting breastfeeding right for you and your baby from the very beginning. It is about solving any problems quickly and easily.

There are many detailed photographs and illustrations that will show you exactly what to do. These pictures are probably the most valuable part of the book. It is always easier to understand breastfeeding by seeing it than by reading about it.

The book has three important subjects: why breastfeeding is best for you; how to get the basics of breastfeeding right, including a simple checklist; breastfeeding problems: causes and solutions.

The same principles that help you get it right from the start will also guide you in treating common problems. Even unusual situations—which are rare in breastfeeding—can be improved or corrected by following these guidelines. If you have a special problem and need more help, on page 203 there is a list of further, more detailed reading and a directory of good resources and organizations in different countries.

We give only information that we are confident about, and that has been well tried and tested. When we make observations and suggestions that are not yet fully supported by research, we point this out.

The reference list at the back of the book gives what we feel are some of the most significant sources in the huge volume of literature used in the preparation of this book. The index will help you find what you need quickly.

Three practical points:

1. We have written this book so that it is appropriate for all those who read English. There are cultural differences in the use and writing of the English language. With one English, one American, and one Scottish author who has spent part of her life in Canada, we hope we have achieved a balance of language. We have chosen one consistent style of spelling. Because our publisher is American, we use American spelling throughout. We hope that non-Americans do not feel excluded by this.

2. Babies are either girls or boys. We acknowledge this by alternating the use of him and her, she and he in different sections of the book.

3. We are using the term health worker to include every trained person a woman may have access to—professional or lay. Where we mean specifically a medical practitioner, we say so.

What This Book Will Do for You

This book will help you get the basics of breastfeeding right, for you and for your baby. It will help you to prevent problems and treat them quickly if they occur.

What we offer does not include the use of drugs or mechanical inventions, such as nipple shields or the regular use of bottles. We do mention a few simple aids, such as spoons, cups, and breast pumps, for use in special situations. Our main purpose, however, is to show you the basics of breastfeeding, which require only you and your baby. Most of the problems women have are a result not knowing these basic principles. You can often work out your own problems if you have the right information. Some problems will need specialist help, but all mothers need to understand the basics first.

This book will help others help you to continue with good breastfeeding. Sometimes it is hard to solve problems on your own. You can share this book with your partner, your helpers, or others who are important to you. It will help them to support you! Many people say it is hard to support breastfeeding when someone they care for is struggling with problems, is exhausted, or is in pain. Understandably they want to take action to help. Sadly, the most common remedy today is to give the baby a bottle, rather than try to solve the real problem.

This book will help you avoid and understand the conflicting advice so commonly given to women. It may contradict much of what you have heard (and may well continue to hear) from family, friends, and health workers. There are reasons for this, which we will explain. *This book will help you to sort out the good advice from the bad.*

This book will give you back a real choice in feeding your baby: *the choice to* *breastfeed well, with pleasure, by avoiding problems or solving them early and successfully. We want every woman to be able to say what one mother recently said about her baby daughter: "She's been a joy—for all of us!"*

Who This Book Is For

This book is for all women, all over the world, who want to know more about feeding their babies. It is for you:

- Whether you have or have not yet decided to breastfeed
- Whether you have or have not yet had a baby
- Whether you are having your first baby, or your second, third, or more
- Whether you have or have not had feeding problems in the past
- Whether you are having one baby, twins, or more
- Whether you are on our own or surrounded by friends and helpers
- Whether you are aged fourteen or forty

It is also for people who want to help, such as:

- Men who want to help but are not sure how
- Family and friends who want to offer their support
- Health workers and their babies, who work with women and babies

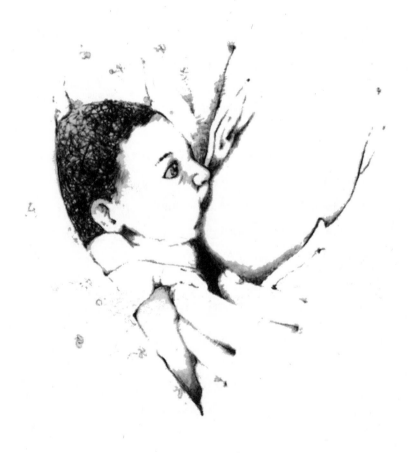

CHAPTER ONE

Why Women Want to Breastfeed

W E do not pretend to be unbiased. Like most women, we believe that breastfeeding is the best way to feed a baby. The evidence is that breastfeeding is good for mothers and best for babies, and no other form of infant feeding has yet been devised that does not have drawbacks.

Best for Babies

What many people don't understand is:

1. Breast milk is perfectly balanced for babies; it has just the right amounts of protein, fat, carbohydrates, minerals and vitamins

2. Breast milk actually changes its composition throughout the day (even through-out each feed!) and over the months, to suit the individual needs of each baby

Most people also know that breastfeeding is the best possible protection against infection and disease. In fact, the more we learn about breastfeeding, the more advantages we see for the baby and the mother. Breastfed babies seem to be protected against some adult diseases, for example, and may even have higher IQs.

In many parts of the world the difference between breastfeeding and bottle feeding is the difference between life and death. Even in countries where bottle feeding is relatively safe, there are still disadvantages in the use of feeding bottles and artificial milk.

For example, it has been shown that breastfeeding is good for:

- The efficiency of the baby's immune system

- The strength of the mother-child relationship

- The eating habits of babies, children, and even adults who have been breastfed

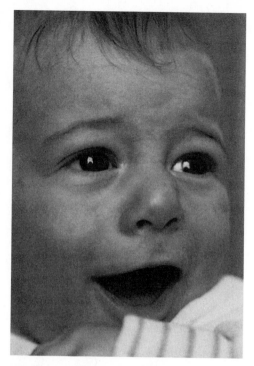

Breastfeeding also seems to decrease the chances of children developing allergies, cancer, Crohn's disease, diabetes, and other problems such as coeliac disease in later life. Many of these diseases are on the increased in industrialized societies. Adults who have been breastfed seem to be less likely to develop arteriosclerosis, and if it does occur, it is likely to be less severe. This area is difficult to research, and studies give few definitive answers. But there are strong indications that these things are true.

Breastfeeding is best for babies.

There are also some studies that suggest that breastfeeding may be good for brain development, for healing the effects of trauma at birth, for children's interpersonal relationships, for children's ability to give comfort, and to comfort themselves, and for children's sleeping patterns. Traditionally, women have used breastmilk to treat their babies' sticky eyes. Some midwives recommend this before using antibiotics. *Artificial feeding provides none of these unique protections. And even in Western countries, babies who are fed artificially have a higher hospital admission rate than babies who are breastfed, especially those who are fully breastfed.*

New information from research done in Sweden suggests that hormones in the baby's digestive system are released by suckling. These hormones help to stimulate the baby's growth and to calm her too. Not only are you feeding your baby, but you are helping her grow and keeping her calm and happy.

Best for Women

Breastfeeding is not only best for babies. It affects women too. Just as in pregnancy it is impossible to separate the mother and baby, so in breastfeeding their physical and emotional welfare are interconnected. A baby who is breastfeeding well is content and grows steadily, and his mother will therefore be more relaxed and happy. Similarly, a relaxed and happy mother is more likely to be able to care well for her baby than an anxious and distressed mother.

For example, women find that when they breastfeed:

- Their wombs contract more quickly after birth.

- The blood loss after childbirth (lochia) flows faster and is completed more quickly.

- They are less likely to become pregnant again soon after birth, especially when breastfeeding is frequently and prolonged.

- The hormones they secrete while breastfeeding make them feel calm.

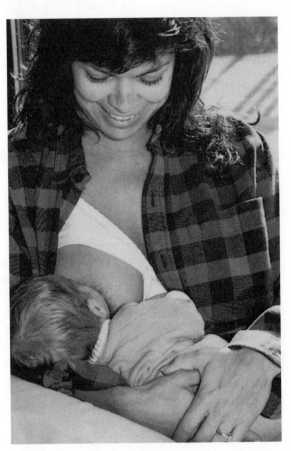

- The hormones make their bodies more efficient while breastfeeding; they don't have to "eat for two," because their bodies conserve energy and use stored energy instead.

- They lose weight more easily, especially around the thighs and buttocks, where fat is usually so hard to shift.

- In later life women who have breastfed seem to be less likely to develop cancer of the breasts, ovaries, and cervix. More research is needed to confirm these effects.

Breastfeeding is best for mothers.

Best for Families

Mothers say that breastfeeding gives them quiet, relaxing times together with their babies throughout the day. If breastfeeding works well, it is pleasurable for mother and baby, and is good for the way a mother and her child feel about themselves and about each other.

Breastfeeding is far more than a way to feed a baby. It is a time when babies and mothers give and receive love. Babies respond not only to the breast milk they take in, but also to the skin-to-skin contact that occurs. Often, crying and distressed babies are comforted by this cuddly contact.

The repeated positive feelings of nurturing and physical closeness are the best possible foundation for a good relationship between mother and baby, and for building the confidence and self-esteem of both. This, in turn, will help promote the development of healthy relationship within the whole family.

Best for Women and Babies with Special Needs

Breastfeeding is best for women and babies, even in special situations, such as having twins or triplets. A woman can produce enough milk to feed more than one baby, and it is often possible to feed two babies at once, once breastfeeding each baby is well established. Many women who must live in circumstances that are far from ideal have discovered breastfeeding to be one thing from which they can draw comfort and support. Breastfeeding well can help a woman gain the confidence to deal with even very difficult circumstances in her life, whether they are physical difficulties or emotional ones.

When the baby needs extra special care, breastfeeding can also help there. It is always hard for parents with small, sick, or premature babies to feel fully involved in their care while they are in the hospital. A mother who expresses her breast milk, and then puts her baby to the breast when she can, is giving her baby a special gift that no one else can. A woman will often say that it involves her in her baby's care and gives her a closeness to her baby that nothing else could. One study has found that premature babies fed with breastmilk were much less likely to develop serious gastrointestinal problems than babies fed on formula milk.

Studies have looked at the benefits of skin-to-skin contact between mothers and their small or sick babies. Often the contact involves the baby nuzzling, or actually feeding, at the breast. Mothers who do this are likely to continue to breastfeed longer than mothers who have not had this opportunity. Their babies gain weight faster and go home from the hospital sooner than babies fed artificial milk.

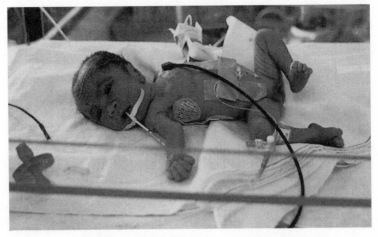

Breastfeeding is best for babies with special needs. Babies who are very small or sick need both the benefits of breast milk and the warm, close contact breastfeeding provides.

Balancing the Benefits and Problems

For each woman, the decision to breast or to bottle feed is a balance between a number of factors. Sometimes these factors conflict. For example, you might believe that breastfeeding is best for your baby, but your sister had serious problems breastfeeding and you are worried the same might happen to you. Or perhaps you want to breastfeed, but you also need, or want, to go back to work soon after your baby's birth. Maybe you are worried about information you have heard about contamination of breast milk due to pollution in our environment. You worry that this might harm your baby, yet, otherwise, you know that breastfeeding is best for your baby. You may want to share responsibility for your baby with your partner, or other friends and family, but can't work out how to do this without using bottles to feed your baby.

Think carefully and weigh the benefits against the hazards before you make a decision. In almost every case, breastfeeding will be by far the best way to feed your baby, and often it will be best for you too. But you need to think through the things that worry you.

Will Breastfeeding Be Difficult For You?

You cannot know this in advance. But the best thing to do is exactly what you are doing: learn as much as you can, find good help, and then begin to breastfeed. Some women have no problems, and most problems that do occur can be treated. This book will help you prevent many of the common problems and provides effective solutions if they do arise.

Can You Combine Breastfeeding and Working?
(see also page 146)

Yes, you can. It is not easy in societies where the workplace is separated from the home, but it can be done. Decisions about whether and when to go back to work outside the home after having a baby are hard. Some women have no choice—they have to return to work because they have to earn enough to support themselves and their family. Others will want to continue to work outside the home because of the sense of satisfaction it gives them, or to continue to develop their careers. Whether you go back to work willingly or unwillingly, you can still continue to enjoy your baby, and to breastfeed. It will help if you think about it beforehand, and plan for your own individual circumstances. You may live close to your work, for example, or you may have a large distance to travel. You may have a supportive partner who can help with childcare at the beginning and the end of the day, or you may be a single parent. You may have a supportive employer, or you may not. There may be good national legislation to protect your rights as a working mother, or you may live in a country (such as the USA) where this is not the case. You may have to go back to work in the early weeks after birth, or you may be able to stay home for several months.

The more time you can be together with your baby during the first few weeks and months, the better for both of you. The best preparation for going back to work is to be breastfeeding without problems. If you have problems and go back to work, it is much harder to keep breastfeeding. Whatever happens, and whenever you go back to work, remember that breastfeeding for even a short time is better for both of you than not breastfeeding at all.

It helps at lot to be in touch with other women who have combined working outside the home with breastfeeding. The challenge can be managed in many different ways. You will get ideas about what may work for you by talking with women who have done it.

Think carefully about all the possibilities. The time you spend thinking creatively and planning carefully ensures that you and your baby can have the solution that is best for you both.

Questions to Ask About Going Back to Work

Can I take paid maternity leave? If so, how will this affect my promotion prospects?

If not, can I take unpaid leave, even for a short while? Again, will this affect my promotion prospects?

Can I work part-time for a while? Will this affect my role and responsibilities, or my promotion prospects?

Can I find good childcare which suits my needs?

Can I breastfeed at lunchtime or on coffee breaks?

Can I take my baby to work for a while?

Can someone bring my baby to me for feeding?

What facilities are there at work for a breastfeeding mother? For example, will you be allowed time to express milk or to feed your baby? Is there a private place to feed or express milk, is there a fridge to store expressed milk, and a clean area to wash your expressing equipment?

Remember you can breastfeed in the evenings and on weekends, while the person caring for your baby feeds expressed breast milk or formula while you are absent.

Policies for women to take maternity leave vary widely from country to country and often even from company to company. Can you take paid maternity leave? If not, are you in a position to take unpaid leave, even for a short while? Can you find good child care close to your workplace, where you could feed at lunchtime? Is your husband, partner, or child carer available to bring the baby to you for feeding through the day? Can you take your baby to work? (If you have a sympathetic employer and colleagues, this is not as impossible as it sounds. In the first few months, many babies simply feed and then sleep quietly.) Can you work part-time for a while? Can you arrange for the time and a quiet place at work to express your milk? Can you arrange to job share? This would mean finding someone to work half-time at your job. One of you could work mornings and the other could work afternoons, or each could work two-and-a-half days a week. Some women who job share look after each others' baby during the time the other is at work.

If none of these solutions are possible, then you might think about cutting down on breastfeeding. The person caring for your baby can give bottles of expressed breast milk or of formula while you are away. You can breastfeed in the mornings, evenings, and on weekends. It is perfectly possible to breastfeed two or three times a day for as long as you want. (See page 146 for more about breastfeeding and working.)

What About Contaminants?

In recent years, newspaper and magazine articles and radio and television programs have warned about the contamination of breastmilk by substances such as pesticides and other chemicals. Some women have chosen not to breastfeed as a result of this information.

All the information we have at the moment suggests that breastmilk is still safer for babies, in spite of this problem. Virtually all studies on this issue stress that the benefits of breastfeeding outweigh the risks of chemical contamination. Stopping breastfeeding would mean that the baby would lose all the health-giving aspects of breastmilk, too.

One reason for our view is that alternative feeds for babies can also contain such contaminants. For example, a study carried out in the UK in 1996 found residues of phthalates in samples of infant formula tested. Another reason is that many studies carried out on dioxins in breastmilk (the chemicals that give most cause for concern) in many countries have shown that their levels are decreasing, probably as a result of moves to decrease the use of chemicals which result in dioxins being released in the environment.

Although we believe that breastfeeding is still safer, this is still a problem which needs to be taken seriously. Many governments have already made changes to help to avoid sources of contamination—for example, stubble burning has been banned in some countries, as have particularly dangerous chemicals. There is little that can be done as an individual to help, however. One factor which might help is not to diet during breastfeeding, as some chemicals stored in the fat in your body are released, as fat stores are mobilized when you diet.

In the long term, society needs to work toward preventing and cleaning up the pollution that caused the contamination in the first place. This will vary from country to country, as the sources of contamination, and the controls in place to prevent them, vary widely. Examples are using lead free fuel, changing industrial processes such as incineration and paper bleaching, working on ways of avoiding huge oil spillages, and finding alternatives to stubble burning.

The World Health Organization has been working on this problem for some years, and there are indications that the situation is improving overall, and that, as we said, levels of chemical contaminants in breastmilk are decreasing.

HIV and AIDS

In recent years, there has been growing concern about the risk of babies becoming infected by the human immunodeficiency virus (HIV) through breast-feeding. HIV is the virus that causes acquired immune deficiency syndrome (AIDS). Some drugs, combined with good care and prompt attention to any illness, can help to improve quality of life and extend the time of survival of a person who has AIDS. However, since there is still no cure for AIDS, it is important that babies are protected as much as possible from HIV infection.

How is the virus transmitted?

HIV is found and can be transmitted in body fluids such as blood, semen, and vaginal secretions. HIV can be transmitted during sexual intercourse, or by sharing injection needles, with someone who has the virus. It can also be passed from a mother who has the virus to her unborn baby during pregnancy or birth, or by breastfeeding. We discuss breastfeeding and HIV transmission more fully below. *It is important to remember that other forms of contact with a person who has the virus, such as touching, hugging or kissing, will not put you at risk of infection.*

Receiving treatment with blood and blood products, such as by blood transfusion or during treatment for haemophilia (a disease that can cause problems with blood clotting), is a possible source of infection. In almost all countries, blood donations are now screened for HIV, and blood products are treated to ensure that if it or other viruses are present, they are inactivated.

HIV can be present in the body for many years without causing AIDS, and many people do not know they have it. If you are concerned that you may have the virus, then talk to a health worker. You may even want to have a blood test. Remember that if you are very recently infected, a blood test may be negative. This is because it takes time for the antibodies to the virus to develop. Most tests are able to detect the antibodies, but not the virus itself. So your health worker may advise you to have another test even if the first one is negative.

What about HIV and breastmilk?

We still have much to learn about the transmission of HIV from mothers to babies through breastmilk, but we do know that babies have become infected this way. As we said above, the most common route for babies to become infected is during pregnancy, labour and birth. In most cases where a mother is HIV positive and her baby becomes infected, it is impossible to tell whether or not the baby became infected in pregnancy, during birth, or after birth, perhaps by breastfeeding.

We know that some babies must have become infected after birth since they were fed by:

- mothers who became infected, after the birth of their baby, by a blood transfusion that was infected with HIV

- mothers who tested negative for HIV while pregnant, but who then showed evidence of infection after birth. They could have been infected during pregnancy, but not yet have developed the antibodies which result in a positive test. Or they may have become infected after the birth

- a wet-nurse who was ill with AIDS

In all of these situations, breastmilk might be especially infective. Infection becomes more likely if mothers are recently infected or are ill with AIDS—at these times, it is easier for the baby to become infected than if the mother has had HIV for some time, and is not ill.

Recent information suggests that if babies are breastfed by a mother who is HIV positive, it is best if they are fed exclusively on breastmilk for the first three months. Giving additional food and fluids seems to increase the risk that the baby will become HIV positive—perhaps because these extra foods and fluids cause some damage to the lining of the baby's gut and reduce the protection that breastmilk gives against infection.

Balancing the risks and benefits

The risk of HIV transmission through breastfeeding is a very important issue, and one we must take seriously. Infection with HIV is life-threatening for the baby. But in some countries, not breastfeeding is also life-threatening. All babies are likely to develop other infections if they are fed a breast milk substitute—and it is very important to keep people with HIV protected from infection as much as possible. So there are no clear or easy answers.

The World Health Organization (WHO), UNICEF and UNAIDS have published guidelines for health workers about this situation, as it is not easy to decide what to do in some circumstances. In environments where safe alternatives to breastfeeding are usually not available, including developing countries, governments and health workers have a serious challenge. WHO is working with them to advise health workers, and women, appropriately.

Our view, based on all the recent evidence and the international guidelines, is as follows:

Women who are certain that they are not infected with HIV, because they have had a negative blood test, or because they have done nothing to expose themselves to a possible source of infection, can breastfeed with confidence.

Women who know they are infected with HIV, and have had a blood test that shows this, should seek the advice of a health worker about breastfeeding. It is now possible to reduce HIV infection rates by giving antiretroviral drugs to a mother during pregnancy (we do not know if the same is true of taking these drugs during breastfeeding, since research is not yet complete). If rates of mother-to-baby infection before birth can be reduced, it makes sense to reduce the risk of infection after birth, too, perhaps by using an alternative to breastfeeding. But this will depend very much on where women live, whether or not they have access to these drugs in pregnancy, and how safe the alternatives to breastfeeding are in their environment. If women do decide to breastfeed, they should breastfeed exclusively—without adding any other food or fluids—for at least three months, and for longer if possible.

Women who think they might be infected with HIV should seek help from a health worker, and think seriously about having a blood test to see whether or not they are infected. In many cases, they will find that they are not infected, that their worries are groundless; they can relax and breastfeed with confidence. If the test is positive, a woman can then work out what to do with the help and support of her health worker. She may be able to use drugs to reduce the risk of transmission during pregnancy. Her baby will be better cared for after birth if health workers know he may be HIV positive, and they will check him regularly. If she chooses an alternative to breastfeeding, her health worker will advise her about the best way to do this, depending on her circumstances. If she chooses to breastfeed, full breastfeeding is better than mixed feeding for the first few months.

If you are worried about being infected with HIV, and have already started to breastfeed, then continue breastfeeding while you seek help and advice from a health worker.

Some women may be anxious about being infected and feel reluctant to tell anyone about their fears. If you feel like this, think carefully. Do you have real grounds to worry about being infected? Consider once again the ways that infection happens which we described at the beginning of this section. If you are generally anxious that you may have 'caught' it, your fears are probably groundless and you should relax. If you have reason to be anxious, about a past blood transfusion before routine testing was introduced, or about transmission during sexual intercourse, or by sharing injection needles, then please think again about talking to a health worker. If you don't, you may go on worrying about yourself and your baby. And your fears may be completely groundless. If you are infected, it will help you and your baby a lot to have the support of the health services.

Whatever you decide to do, please do not be tempted to give your baby a breastmilk substitute 'just in case'. Babies need breastmilk, and they should have a breastmilk substitute only if it is really necessary. If you want to breastfeed your baby, the only thing that should make you stop and think is if you are DEFI-NITELY HIV positive. Even then, your decision will depend very much on your personal circumstances.

Choosing to Breastfeed

Despite the fact that most women know that breastfeeding is best for their babies, some decide not to breastfeed, and others stop after a short time. When we look at some of the problems that women face when feeding their babies, this is not hard to understand.

A woman who chooses not to breastfeed always has reasons for doing so, which usually include:

• Breastfeeding does not appeal to her or is distasteful to her.

• She believes that breastfeeding is inconvenient and that bottle feeding is much easier.

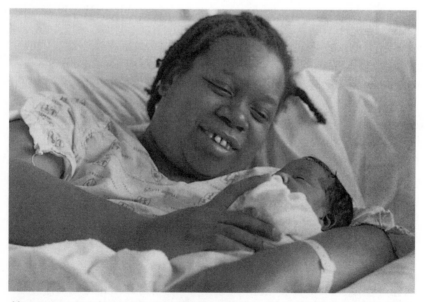

Many women look forward the breastfeeding as a time of special closeness with their babies and something only they can give.

- She plans to go back to work outside the home soon after the baby is born and feels it is too difficult to work and also breastfeed.

- She believes that artificial milks are just as good as—perhaps even better than—breast milk.

When a woman finds the idea of breastfeeding unappealing, it may be a result of her own or other people's experiences, or it may be because she associates breastfeeding with something distasteful. She may, for example, be shy about exposing her breasts or dislike her body. But women in cultures where modesty is prized breastfeed, even in public places, without exposing their breasts. And many women who have learned to dislike or distrust their bodies, but who have been willing to breastfeed for all the benefits it has for their babies, have found a measure of comfort and pleasure in breastfeeding they had never thought possible.

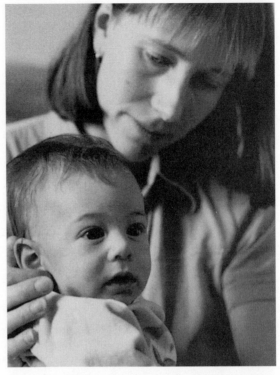

Some women feel a bit anxious at the idea of breastfeeding. This may be because of things others have said or negative experiences they have had.

A woman who decides not to breastfeed because she believes bottle feeding is equal to breastfeeding and is easier is usually unaware of the difficulties, hazards, and practical drawbacks of bottle feeding.

A woman who plans to go back to work outside the home while her baby is very young and believes it is not possible both to do this and to breastfeed needs information that it is possible to do both, for her own benefit and for her baby's.

Some women today, because of their experience and the attitudes of those around them, believe that breastfeeding will not suit their ways of life. They believe that bottle feeding is a good choice for themselves and their babies.

It is important that every woman makes a free choice about how to feed her baby. She cannot do this unless she has full information about breastfeeding and bottle feeding, breast milk and artificial milk. A woman who chooses not to breastfeed might want to ask herself, Why do I not want to breastfeed? Are my reasons sound? Can some of the problems be overcome?

If women found breastfeeding easy, *if* our culture did not lead some women to regard the workings of their bodies with uneasiness, and *if* artificial substitutes were not so heavily advertised and easily available, *then* women would truly have free choice.

Women are often prevented from doing what they would like to do by three things:

1. **Misinformation** they are given by others, which creates bad habits and leads to breastfeeding problems

2. **Lack of skilled support**, especially in the first days and weeks

3. **Practical difficulties** they can't solve

You can see that the problems of breastfeeding, which are common, arise largely from social, not individual causes.

It is not a woman's fault if she chooses not to breastfeed, or if she stops in the first weeks or months. It is often the fault of the culture in which we live. Women are simply not being given the accurate information and skilled support they need to carry on.

Western cultures look on breasts mainly for sexual pleasure, and women often find it hard to expose their breasts to feed their babies. This is in spite of the fact that breastfeeding often exposes less of the breast than normal beachwear and many women now sunbathe and swim topless. Some men in Western society also find it hard for their partners to breastfeed while other people are around. Some even feel jealous and threatened by the special closeness their babies have with their mothers at their mothers' breasts. This is hard to deal with, because the feelings are so deep rooted. It is a fact, however, that babies need breasts, and they need them to be available when they are hungry, not just when it is convenient for older people.

Women should not feel guilty for choosing to avoid or to solve their problems by bottle feeding. Sadness or anger might be more natural responses, for women have not had the help they need to learn and maintain this essential skill.

Successful breastfeeding must become a real choice for women today. When it does many more people will gain confidence in the fact that women's bodies work, and that babies are the best judges of their own food intake.

A Formula for Trouble

Try adding together

a difficult-to-cope-with, unhappy baby
(a common result of difficult breastfeeding)

with

a new mother who feels unsure of how to care for a baby
(what new mother who has little experience of babies and little support from experienced mothers isn't unsure of herself?)

with

the demands of an already tiring life
(what parent of a young child isn't usually tired and often dealing with long hours of work in or away from the home?)

and you get

the perfect recipe for breastfeeding failure!

add to that

the fact that many women today are single parents
(trying valiantly to do alone what traditionally was the job of a large, extended family)

plus

the fact that much advice women get is inaccurate or discouraging

plus

the unease some people feel with breasts and breastfeeding
(and it's hard not to feel this, given our culture's obsession with breasts as sex objects)

And you get *a sense of the seriousness and widespread nature of the problem.*

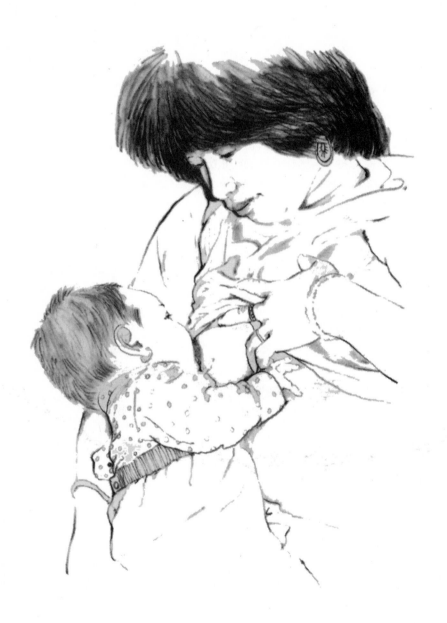

CHAPTER TWO

Starting to Breastfeed: Getting the Basics Right

Before You Begin—Finding Helpers

Finding good helpers is one of the most important things you can do. It might also be one of the hardest.

All women who breastfeed their new babies can benefit from help, especially in the first three to four weeks. Even if you find breastfeeding easy from the beginning, you will need help to allow you time apart from the baby to catch up on your sleep. Whether this is your first baby or your sixth, you need to think about who is going to help you. Try to choose your helpers before your baby is born.

Note: If you don't have good support, this does not mean you will fail, or that you should choose to bottle feed. But it helps enormously to have support.

You will need three things from your helpers:

1. ***Good emotional support*** on an ongoing basis while you work on getting breastfeeding established or on solving problems.

2. ***Real practical help*** with household tasks, such as shopping, cooking, cleaning, and caring for your older children.

3. ***Skilled assistance*** if you have difficulty getting it right or if you develop problems.

Helpers can be your friends, husband or partner, family, midwife, doctor, health visitor, nurse, lactation consultant, or breastfeeding support group. Women who have breastfed well or a nutritionist may also be able to help. If you cannot find good help, look at the resources listed at the back of this book. These organizations may be able to put you in touch with someone nearby.

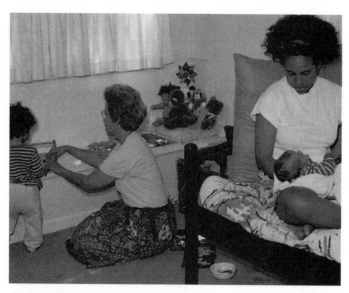

A helper can take care of the house, cook, and assist with older children. She can make things a bit easier for you, so that you can concentrate on getting breastfeeding established and enjoying your baby.

Before you turn to someone for help, make sure whoever you ask is as interested in breastfeeding as you are. If one of his or her first solutions is to try bottle feeding, that person is not the right person to ask. If this happens to you, find someone else.

It is possible that one person alone (even the most loving and attentive husband or partner) will not be able to help you in every way necessary. It is unlikely that he or she will be available every time you need someone or be skilled at solving a physical problem, such as the position of the baby at the breast. But this person's emotional encouragement will be a great help, and together you may be able to resolve the problem or find additional help.

Usually a partner, friends, and family are good sources of help for emotional and practical support. You might want to ask your mother, or another relative who supports your breastfeeding, or a friend to stay for the first few days to help.

If you ask someone to come and stay and help, then let him or her do just that. Don't be tempted to look after that person as a guest. And don't let him or her play with the baby while you do the dishes, either. This time is for you and your baby to get to know each other. Ask only someone you feel very relaxed with (and this may not necessarily be your mother, no matter how much she loves you).

Remember that because bottle feeding was common until the last few years, many older women did not breast feed. Your mother and your mother-in-law may have bottle fed. Some will not be supportive of breastfeeding, simply because their experience was different. Do think carefully before you decide where to turn for help. The last thing you need to hear as your work on getting breastfeeding right at 2:00 a.m. is, "Why don't we just try a bottle?"

If your partner is not supportive, then ask a friend you see often or who lives nearby to help. A woman who has breastfed well herself is an invaluable resource.

A mother-to-mother support group, such as La Leche League (in the U.S. and many other countries), Nursing Mothers Council (the U.S.), the National Childbirth Trust, Association of Breastfeeding Mothers, and the Breastfeeding Network (in the United Kingdom), or the Nursing Mothers Association (in Australia), can often provide this sort of support. See the listing of resources at the back of this book (page 203) for how to contact them.

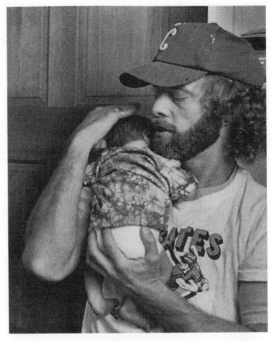

The father can be a tremendous help with the new baby and your greatest support during the first weeks, as you both learn to cope with little sleep and adjust your lives to this new person who needs so much care and attention.

A Word About Fathers or Partners

The father of your baby can be your best support for breastfeeding. He may enjoy watching and helping you and the baby be physically close and loving. Or he may find it challenging and uncomfortable, and he may feel left out or threatened by how close you and the baby are.

Because of the complex issues of sexuality and breastfeeding in many cultures, some men have ambivalent feelings about breastfeeding, of which they may not even be aware. Your baby's father may want to support you, yet find it hard when you need to feed in front of other people. He may like the idea of breastfeeding, but find the practicalities hard to take. Or he may be supportive while it is going well, but find it hard to watch you get sore and tired if you have problems.

It will be helpful if your husband or partner understands that in spite of the cultural attitudes that are not always supportive of breastfeeding, it is by far the best thing for your baby and for you. In the long run it will also be the best thing for him, as his baby will be healthier and family relationships will be better and stronger.

Some men want to share in feeding their baby, and some couples feel feeding is an experience they want the father to share. It is important to understand that doing this in the early weeks could undermine the success of breastfeeding. They also need to know that artificial milk is not as good for a baby as breast milk (and

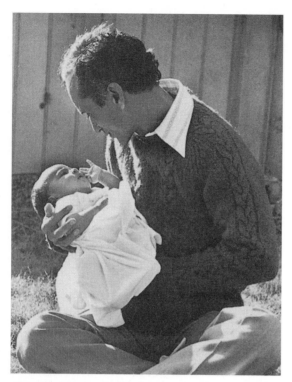

Sometimes the greatest help you can get is some time alone without your baby. A father also needs times alone with his baby.

it's more expensive). After breast-feeding is going well and is easy for both mother and baby, you can express your milk, store it in a bottle, and have someone else feed your baby. This is necessary if you must be apart from the baby when she needs to feed. And that is a time when a father can step in to help.

Men can share in many ways, but feeding is best left to mothers and babies. Fathers can cuddle, comfort, bathe, and change babies, and they can enjoy watching you feed the baby. They can have lots of loving contact, and the baby needs their love and affection.

A Special Message to Fathers and Partners

The two most important things you can do in the first weeks are:

• Give loving support and encouragement to your breastfeeding partner

• Take over more of the daily running of the household.

Your baby's mother needs to be able to focus her attention on the baby and herself in the early weeks. She needs a partner who participates fully. Breast-feeding is the simplest and best way to feed a baby, but it is not always easy at the beginning.

Your partner might like a gentle massage. A breastfeeding mother's neck and shoulders can get tense. Give practical help whenever you can. Try offering a drink (a breastfeeding mother can forget how thirsty she is). Suggest that you cuddle the baby for a few minutes so she can take a bath or shower or just go to the bathroom. Perhaps she'd like you to brush her hair.

It's the little things that you do on a daily basis that make all the difference. Do your share of changing your baby's diapers/nappies. Keep up with the laundry, the dishes, tidy up the room where your baby and partner spend most of their time. And, please find the time each day to sit down with her and give your partner some of your time to listen to her feelings. As demanding as these early weeks are for *all* of you, a mother can still feel lonely, anxious or blue. Her hormones are rapidly changing, and getting less sleep than usual doesn't help.

When the baby is crying, try picking her up and comforting her, see if her diaper (nappy) needs changing, and change it if it does. Babies cry for more reasons than hunger. They have all the feelings adults have, and your baby is still adapting to life outside the womb. Babies don't come with an instruction manual. You have to learn as you go along, just as mothers do. You will learn to understand your baby's needs by responding to her facial expressions and sounds, including her different types of crying, with interest and tenderness. That is something you can do from the very beginning. And, in that way, you will become extremely close to your baby, even though you cannot breastfeed.

Finding Skilled Assistance

Finding skilled assistance might be difficult because of the reasons discussed on pages 147-148. Many health workers do not really understand breastfeeding, even if they are supportive. So be creative if you need to, and be persistent.

In some places midwives or pediatricians are specializing in breastfeeding. Some are even setting up special services for breastfeeding mothers in addition to the normal postnatal services. Public health nurses in some locations may be helpful in the United States, where there is no organized postpartum care for mothers and babies; in many parts of the country any woman can ask for a home visit from a public health nurse. Usually such a visit is free. To find this person may not be easy, because public health care is organized differently in different localities. First try calling your local social services department listed in the front of your phone book. If there is no service available, then ask what agency does provide home visits.

In the United States, Australia and several other countries, a new profession has evolved: the lactation consultant. These are women who have a variety of backgrounds but wish to concentrate on helping women to breastfeed successfully. Some are employed in hospitals; others work independently in the community. See page 203 for help in finding one.

All the guidelines we have given in this section about finding help also apply to finding professional help. You might also want to talk to other women, and find out who has been helpful to them.

If there is no one nearby who has real skill, then find a health worker who is concerned and supportive, and take a copy of this book with you. Together you should be able to work it out.

Taking Care of Yourself

Having a new baby is likely to be the most demanding experience you will ever have. Along with discovering the real rewards and joys of this time, you will find that you are very tired. This is due in part to the inevitable nights of broken sleep and early waking.

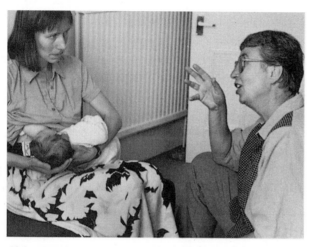

Make sure the person you choose to help you breastfeed is interested in breastfeeding and will take the time to work with you and your baby.

Don't be surprised that you don't have as much energy as you are used to. Most of your energy is going toward caring for your baby. This experience is valuable and rewarding, but you might find that you cannot work, at home or at your job, with the same enthusiasm as you did before. You now have an extra, time-consuming job to do, and your life will have to change.

Some magazines and books will tell you that you can still do it all—the Superwoman myth. This is not true. You might be able to do it for a while, but in the long term your own health and the happiness of those around you will suffer. Find ways of cutting back the other demands in your life, at least for a while. Doing less housework, or getting help with the basic tasks, is one way of adjusting. Many couples find that work in the home must be shared more evenly once they have a baby.

Make sure you take some time for yourself at least once a day. Having someone care for your baby for a short time while you take a restful bath or walk or read quietly can make all the difference. You can't expect anyone to read your mind and know your needs (much as it would be nice, especially when you're tired). Asking for help from others may not be easy for you; this is the time to learn how.

You might be surprised and dismayed to find that you are feeling very emotional and your moods are swinging. *Why do I feel like crying, when I am happy to be a mother?* or *"I shouldn't be feeling bad; I have a healthy baby."* The first weeks after birth are deeply influenced by changing hormones. Your body goes through a tremendous shift from its pregnant state to breastfeeding and mothering, particularly if this is your first baby. In addition, you might well have a mix of strong emotions, especially if the birth did not go the way you'd hoped, or if you found the experience traumatic. It's quite amazing how easily most women make this enormous shift to becoming a mother, but it always takes time. Many women feel weepy or melancholy, usually about the third day after birth, when the breasts become active. This is when you might want extra support; although help and support over the early days and weeks will almost always be welcome.

A new mother needs a balance of enough support and enough privacy (time with just her baby, or with her partner and her baby) and very few are fortunate enough to get it. Many find they have too many visitors but not enough help. Others have lots of time alone with the baby because their partner has gone back to work, but they have no help. Many new mothers, on a natural high from at last holding their new baby, can't sleep at all the first couple of nights. They feel so full of energy they spend it cooking, cleaning, making phone calls, only to crash with exhaustion the day their milk comes in. Many midwives and experienced mothers wisely suggest that a new mother stay in her nightclothes or bathrobe for the first week or two, just to remind herself—and everyone around her—that she is not ready to resume her hectic life.

Everything you do for your baby, especially the things you do often in a day, such as picking her up or changing her diaper, teaches your baby about you and her world. She learns about the world mostly from your behavior, through your touch and the feeling of love and care you give her. This makes it all the more important to take good care of yourself and to *treat yourself as if you are very special and worthwhile, because you are.*

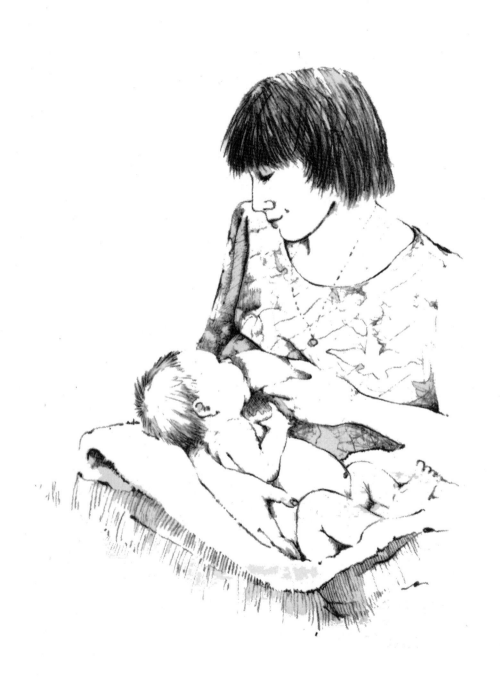

CHAPTER THREE

How Breastfeeding Really Works: The Basics

Breastfeeding without problems depends on getting the physical aspects right. Ideally, this means getting it right from the first feed.

☆

We will describe, and show you in photographs and drawings, exactly how to go about getting breastfeeding right.

We define breastfeeding as right if it is free of problems for you and your baby. We do not intend the word *right* to imply that there is only one way to breastfeed or that you have failed if you encounter difficulties. There are as many ways of breast-feeding as there are mothers and babies, and you will develop your own style, just as you would if you were danc-ing; but you need to know the steps first before you can add your own variations.

It is usually not difficult to get breastfeeding right—in fact, you and your baby may find it really easy—but you will need a bit of practice, and you may need the help and support of other people. Remember that many prob-lems last only a week or two,

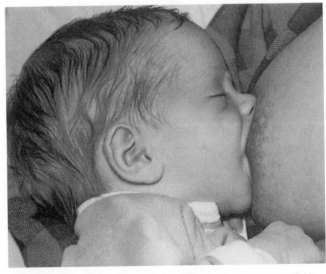

This baby, one of twins, was having difficulty at the breast until his mother learned how to get positioning just right. His brother, who was larger at birth, had no trouble; but like many small babies, positioning was critically important for this little boy. Here, at 3 ½ weeks, he is on the breast well for the very first time. His mother remarked on the difference in his behavior (he was much happier!) after just this one good feed.

and then you and your baby can go on to enjoy months of satisfying breast-feeding.

Some people may think it is unnecessary to go into such detail on these points. But women today didn't learn about breastfeeding by seeing while growing up. Few older women know how to do it right. Many health workers have never learned the techniques of breastfeeding. Most of us need to relearn the practicalities of breastfeeding. Maybe in thirty or forty years' time, so many women will have learned about breastfeeding that a book to teach the techniques will be unnecessary, but that time is not with us yet.

Remember that you will need to practice to get it right. Think about how you learned to walk. It took practice and time; you didn't get it together all at once. You were clumsy at first. You fell sometimes. But you didn't criticize yourself because you didn't get it right the first time. You simply kept practicing, and one day you discovered you could do it easily.

Breastfeeding is a combination of instinct, reflex, and learning. For instance, you have an instinct to put your baby to your breast, and your baby has a reflex to open her mouth. Beyond that, you have to learn what to do with your breast and your baby, and your baby has to learn what to do with her mouth and jaws.

It's like dancing: the two of you may like each other and like the rhythm of the music, but not know the steps to the dance. At first you may get tangled up every time you try, and have to laugh at yourselves. But once you get it right, you are a single unit: you move smoothly, without having to think about it, like one body. And although it can be difficult to learn, it is often fun to practice.

Or breastfeeding can be compared to learning to drive a car. You have to get the details right, in the right sequence, before you can go anywhere without stalling constantly.

It will pay off if you take time and pay careful attention until breastfeeding is going smoothly. When you have learned to drive or to dance, you often wonder what all the fuss was about—but without the fuss, you probably never would have got it right. Once breastfeeding is established, without problems, it will be easy to enjoy both your baby and the rest of your life.

Simple does not always mean easy. What we offer is simple, but it may take time. Once you and your baby get it right, however, you will never forget it. You will add your own variations as you get more confident and as your baby grows, just as you do in developing your own style of dancing or driving.

You can use the information we provide here whether you are starting from your first feed or working on solving problems.

The basic principles we describe are the same at all stages of breastfeeding and for mothers and babies of all ages (although they are most important in the early days and weeks), and whether you are having your first or fourth baby. They are also the same if you have more than one baby to feed or if your baby is small or sick or active or passive.

You will need to prepare for feeding. Quiet surroundings are very helpful in the first two weeks, as you and your baby learn about each other. Some women find that during this time they are easily distracted by visitors with whom they are not entirely comfortable, or even by the radio or television. Others find that by putting on some calming music helps. Once you are quiet and comfortable, focus on your baby, not on what is going on around you.

Take the time you need to get breastfeeding right at the start; it will be easier later if you do. If you can arrange to have extra help in the house at this time, from your husband or partner, family member, or close friend, then do. But make sure it is someone with whom you feel comfortable; otherwise the help will cause more problems than it is worth. And don't be too worried about keeping the house tidy for a while. A happy, healthy baby and a few precious moments of quiet for yourself are more important than a tidy house.

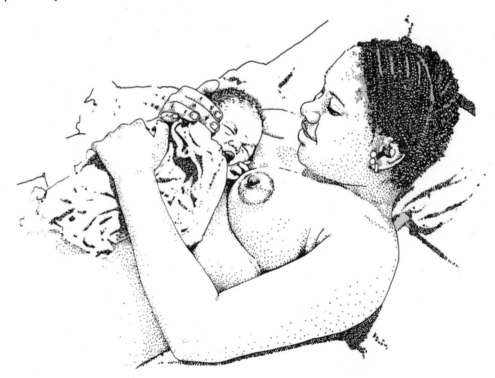

Breastfeeding Your Baby for the First Time

Breastfeeding for the first time—in fact, for the first few days or weeks, until it is easy—is best done when you, your baby, your partner, and your helpers are all calm.

Getting feeding right needs patience and quiet surroundings. It is good to feed soon after delivery, but it does not have to happen immediately. In fact, many babies and many mothers are not ready to feed right after birth; they both need some time to adjust to what has just happened. Hold your baby close after birth if you can, and let her nuzzle at your breasts. If she is eager to feed, she will try to do so. If not, don't try to persuade her until you have calm, quiet time and help to get it right.

After a normal birth, it is probably best to wait until after your placenta (after-birth) is out, your stitches are done (if you need any), and you can move more freely. This will probably be within the first hour after birth. In the meantime, you can keep your baby in your arms and concentrate on enjoying her; you needn't think about breastfeeding until you have a bit of quiet and privacy. When you are ready for breastfeed her, ask for the help of a midwife, nurse, or family member.

There should be no reason for your baby and you to be separated. You can take your time to bring your new baby to your breast. A baby who has not been affected by medication (from pain-relieving drugs in labour) will probably be very alert and may want to feed quite soon. But many healthy babies take an hour or more to want to feed. Your baby may also be quite tired, even stunned, from the journey and just want to rest skin-to-skin—cuddled up close. Just having your baby near your breast has the added benefit of causing a release of hormones that contract your uterus more efficiently. Remember that both you and your baby have just worked very hard, and your bodies will need to recover. Many women like to lie down for the first feed, especially if they have stitches from an episiotomy or have had a cesarean. Some babies will be sleepy and need encouragement to feed for the first days, especially if they are small or if their mothers were given medication during labor.

After an epidural or spinal anesthetic, you will still be awake and able to hold your baby. After a spinal, you may need to lie flat for a few hours to prevent a severe headache. You should be able to feed your baby whenever you and he are ready. However, you may need some help changing position if you are still numb.

If you have had a cesarean section, you can still cuddle and feed your baby soon after delivery, though you will need help. You will have to lie in bed for the first hours, but will probably be encouraged to get up and move around soon, to promote healing.

After a general anesthetic, ask for your baby to be given to you as soon as you waken. A helper can put your baby to your breast, at least for a cuddle, even if you are not fully awake. You can learn how to feed her once you have recovered from the anesthetic. In the meantime you and she will have had time together, and she may have even had a chance to feed, and your breasts will have been stimulated to start making milk.

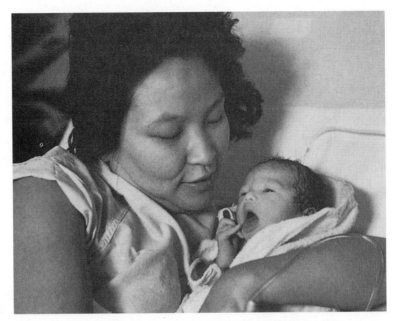

After a cesarean birth you can cuddle and hold your baby almost immediately. Do ask for help to breastfeed for the first few times.

If you have given birth to more than one baby, then you can still cuddle and feed, but probably just with one baby at a time. Your partner or helper can share by cuddling the other baby or babies.

If your baby is taken to the intensive or special care nursery, then you can still stimulate your breast to produce milk soon after delivery. Go see your baby and, if you can, touch or hold her as soon as possible; this will help you and also help your milk supply. Then ask for help in expressing your milk (see pages 86-91 about expression).

Express in the first few hours after birth, and then every three hours or so, regularly, until you can feed your baby. Ask to hold her, or at least touch and stroke her, before you express, as this will help your milk to flow.

Remember that even if your baby does not feed for some time after birth—even days or weeks—but needs intravenous fluids or tube feeding, she will still be able to feed from your breasts when she is well enough. The important thing is to keep your breasts stimulated, so that when she can feed, you have plenty of milk. If you have trouble doing this, try not to worry. Once she is well enough to feed from your breasts, her feeding will soon stimulate your milk (see pages 98-102 for more information on babies who need special care).

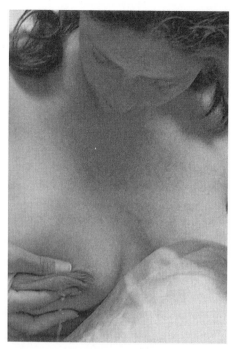

If for any reason your baby cannot breastfeed, start to express your milk so that you baby can still have it.

Before you start any breastfeed, remember that like any meal, you first need to prepare it. The more careful the preparation, the better the food.

Here is a simple way of relaxing.

Before you begin to feed, take three quiet, slow breaths, focusing your full attention on the sensation of simply breathing in and breathing out.

Listen to the sound of the air as it passes down the back of your throat.

Feel your chest and abdomen expand the way a round balloon fills, as the air enters and fills your body, bringing with it the calm you need.

Imagine your breath is your best friend, one who is always there for you, always ready to soothe you when you are tired or stressed.

It is especially important to calm yourself before you try to help your baby if she is crying or upset. It takes only a few seconds. Then, when you are calm, take the time to comfort her. If you cannot calm her, have someone else take her and comfort her. Do this before you try to put her to your breast. It really makes a difference.

To get breastfeeding right, you first need to understand three important aspects:

1. *The way you and your baby are positioned during feeding*

2. *How your body works to produce and release milk*

3. *How the composition of your milk changes in the course of a single feed*

These points are described in detail in the next sections.

Position Matters

Good positioning means getting yourself and your baby into comfortable, effective body positions. When you learn to drive a car, you need to be sitting comfortably in the driver's seat, hands on the wheel and feet on the pedals. You *could* reach the pedals and the wheel by stretching your legs and arms if the seat was too far back from the pedals and wheel or tilted back too far. But it would not be comfortable, effective, or safe, and you would be bound to run into problems.

Or imagine you are learning to type. It's much easier to sit in a good position, so that your body and arms are comfortable. If you are well positioned on a comfortable chair, you will get less tired while typing, and you'll be more accurate too.

Learning to breastfeed is just the same. You may be able to do it if one or both of you is in an awkward position, but it is a recipe for problems in the long run. It's worth the effort to get positioned correctly right from the beginning.

Remember that mothers and babies, everywhere, always have to learn to breastfeed. Like driving a car, typing, or any other skill, some of us learn faster than others. And with breastfeeding there are two of you learning together!

Remember too that for breastfeeding to work well, it does not matter what size your baby is or what shape your nipples are. *Babies don't nipple feed; they breastfeed.*

It doesn't matter how small or big your breasts or nipples are. They are the right size. You can still breastfeed well if you have inverted nipples, although you will need skilled help at first (see pages 91-92).

The information given here is especially for mothers of new babies. Most women find that after they and their babies learn about breastfeeding, they can do it in almost any position, anywhere, at any time. For some it comes easily, straightaway. But at first, for many women, it requires concentration, patience, and practice while learning.

Getting Positioning Right

You need to think about three things as you learn to get positioning right. These are:

1. **Your posture:** Whatever position you are in, whether you are sitting up or lying down, ask yourself when you start, Am I truly comfortable? It is hard to feed your baby well if your back, neck, or shoulder is strained, your arm tired, or your bottom hurts.

2. **The shape of your breast:** Ask yourself, Is the way I am sitting or lying, or what I am doing with my hands, changing the natural shape of my breast?

3. **How you hold your baby:** Ask yourself, Am I holding my baby's body close enough to me? Can he reach my breast comfortably, without having to make an effort?

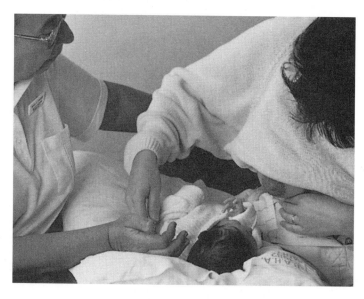

4. **How your baby takes your breast:** Ask yourself, Is he able to take a good mouthful of my breast without having to pull on my nipple?

Your helper must be sitting in a comfortable position alongside you to give you the greatest assistance.

A Note to Helpers If you are a helping, ask yourself, Where am I in relation to this mother and her baby? If you are not in a comfortable position yourself, you may not be able to give the time it takes to help her. Your discomfort may distract you, and she may pick up on your feelings and be ill at ease.

Your Posture

From the very first feed, try not to forget *yourself* in the excitement of putting your baby to your breast. It's still the same as in pregnancy and birth. Whatever you do affects your baby—and the better you look after yourself, the happier you baby will be.

Your body needs to be in a posture where you can hold your baby's body tucked in close to you, and in which your breast does not pull away from her mouth as she feeds.

This means that if you are sitting, you need to be upright, not leaning backward. Look at the pictures here: look at how the woman's breast shape and the directions of her nipple change as she sits upright, as compared to leaning back

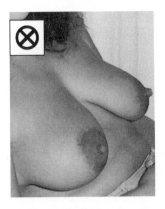
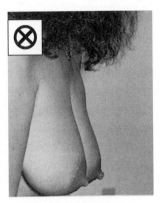
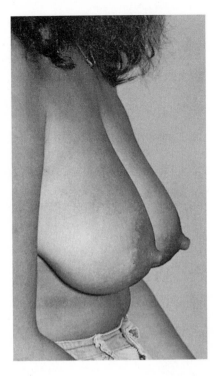

The way you sit (or lie) affects the angle of your breasts and therefore the amount of breast your baby can take.

In the first photograph above (left) the woman is leaning back and her nipple points upward.

In the photograph above (right) she leans too far forward and her nipple points downward.

In this photograph, she is sitting up with her back straight and her breast is in good position for the baby to take.

in the chair. You baby will not be able to get as good a mouthful of your breast if you lean back. Your breast should never be stretched or pulled in the process of feeding, and you should never try to push it out of shape. Remember to bring the baby to your breast, not to twist your body to take your breast to the baby. As your baby gets bigger, you could even turn your body a little away from the baby to leave space for her.

Start by getting yourself into a body position in which you feel comfortable. There are a variety of possible positions: you and your baby will work out the ones that are good for both of you. You will probably use different positions at different times. A few suggestions are:

- **Try sitting in a straight-backed chair if you have one.** This chair should allow your feed to be flat on the floor and your lap flat or your knees just slightly higher than your lap. Do not try sitting in a rocking chair to feed until you and your baby have established a happy feeding relationship. Babies do love and need to be rocked; but save the rocking chair for non-feeding times. It's very hard to sit up straight in a rocking chair and your breasts tend to flatten when you rock back.

- **If you do not have a simple straight-backed chair, you can use an arm-chair or sofa.** But be sure to tuck pillows down behind your back—lower back, upper back, and shoulders, as in the picture on page 37—to support you in an upright position. Many big chairs are deep, and you will need several pillows, cushions, folded blankets, or rugs tucked around you before your back will be straight and your feet flat on the floor.

- **Try sitting on the edge of your bed.** You will have nothing behind your back for support, but you can easily lean slightly forward with your feet on the floor. Use a footstool or books under your feet if the bed is too high. If you are using a hospital bed, you may need to rest your feet on a chair. Put some pillows on your lap to support both your baby and your arms until you get used to this position.
  Note: Be especially careful when you choose to feed sitting up in bed. It can be done, but it is more difficult to get truly upright when your legs are stretched out in front of you. Tuck pillows behind your back. If you have to be in bed it is probably better to feed lying down.

- **You can lie on your side.** This is especially good if you have just given birth and are in bed, have a sore bottom, or have had a cesarean. You can lie anywhere comfortable; your bed, a long sofa, or on the floor.

For this, you will probably need help with the first few feeds, both to lie down comfortably and to position your baby. One you are lying down, you can really use only one arm to help yourself with feeding, as you will lie on or support your weight with the other, so you need someone to put the baby exactly where you want her.

Lying on your side you can choose to feed from either your lower breast (the one closest to the surface you are lying on) or your upper breast. To use the upper breast, you will need to support yourself slightly up on your elbow and turn your upper body so you are leaning over your baby, or let your breast fall into her mouth. Or place your baby up on pillows so that she is level with your breast. Look at the picture on page 37 to see how to do it. Note especially the support from pillows, cushions, and blankets that is needed to keep you and your baby close together when you are lying down.

You may wish to lie with your head and back supported a bit higher than your hips and legs are, like the woman in the picture. If you are in a hospital bed, you can ask someone to raise the back of the bed so your upper body is at a slight angle. At home some big cushions or pillows would have the same effect.

- **It's important to avoid distorting the natural shape of your breast whenever you start to feed.** Distorting the shape can happen in two ways: by poor posture, or by putting your hand or even just your fingers on your breast, in

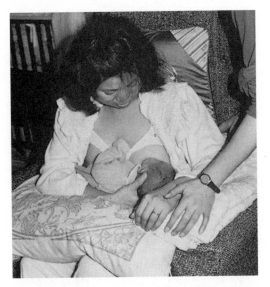

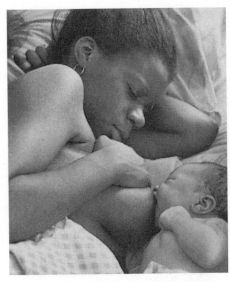

You can breastfeed in an armchair or soft couch—BUT first tuck pillows or cushions down behind your back to support yourself upright. Placing another pillow or two on your lap, so that your baby is supported at the height of your breast takes strain off your shoulders and back.

Lying on your side is also a good way to feed. It may be the only comfortable position for a few days if you have had a cesarean or have a spinal headache and need to remain lying down.

This woman is feeding from the upper breast. To do this she has placed her baby on a thick, firm cushion which supports her body completely and frees her mother's arm.

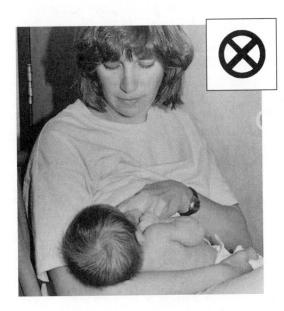

This woman is sitting upright and supporting her baby at the height of her breast (by crossing one knee over the other and resting her forearm on her thigh). What is wrong with this picture?

She has placed the baby's head in the crook of her arm, as if she were bottle feeding (which means that to feed, her baby must pull her breast to the side). Instead, she needs to place the baby a few inches down her forearm.

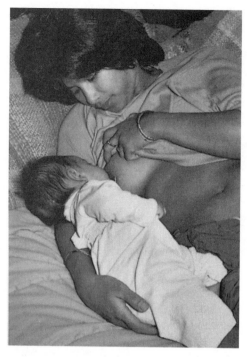

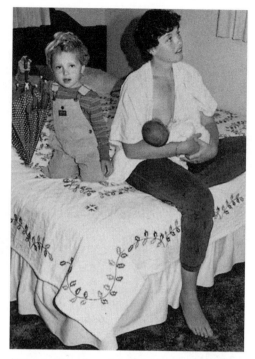

Lying on your side can be an easy way to breastfeed and nap at the same time once you and your baby have learned how to do it.

To breastfeed well in this position, remember to tuck your baby close in to your body (her entire body against yours) and have her head level with your breast so that she does not have to reach for or pull on it. Some mothers find it helpful to tuck the end of a pillow under their ribs, to raise their breast a little off the bed.

You can sit on the edge of the bed to feed, but make sure at least one foot is flat on the floor (putting something under your feet to raise them if you need to). Also remember to keep your back straight and have your baby's head at the height of your breast.

This woman's breasts are low; her baby can lie on her arm and her arm can rest on her thigh without her having to bend her back.

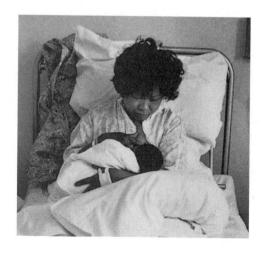

Breastfeeding while sitting up in bed is difficult. If you do this, then have something firm behind to support you sitting upright.

This mother's breasts are high. She needs a pillow under the baby to bring the baby to the right height, so that she does not need to carry the baby's weight in her arms, shoulders, and back.

any way that changes its natural shape—pulling it away from the baby, for example, or trying to push it in. See page 46 [Some important information on Supporting your Breast] to learn how to support your breast. Everything has to do with the relationship between the baby's mouth and your breast. You will get this from us over and over again, because that is core of good breast-feeding.

- **You don't need a chair, sofa, or bed.** You can sit on the floor with your back straight, your legs crossed (as in the photograph on page 40) or in the tailor position (where you sit with your knees open and your feet together). You can put pillows in the hollow between your knees. It is easier if you have a wall behind you. Do keep your back straight.

Experiment with different postures, and try them out to see how they feel for you before you put your baby to your breast. When you read our descriptions in the next section of the positions your baby should be in, you will see why your own posture matters so much.

In summary, the important principles of your posture to get right are:

1. **Make yourself comfortable.** Your body needs to be well supported, so you can hold your baby close to your breast for half an hour or more without your arms getting too tired. If you are comfortable and well-supported you will not have to use any extra effort to hold your baby, and you will not get back, shoulder, or neck tension.

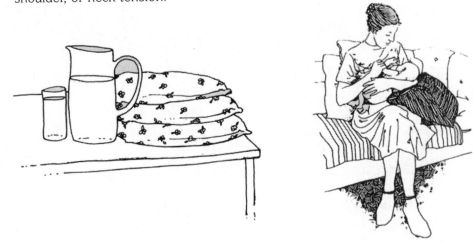

2. **Make sure you are not leaning back**—so that your breasts are not pulled away from your baby and out of his mouth while he tries to feed—or hunched over.

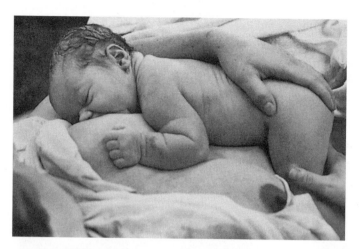

If necessary, you can feed your baby while lying on your back. This is not always easy—it may be difficult for the baby to take enough of your breast and may not stimulate your milk supply enough. It is not recommended for most women.

This mother must temporarily lie on her back to feed, so she drapes here newborn baby's body over hers, and makes sure that the baby takes not only the nipple but a lot of breast tissue in his mouth.

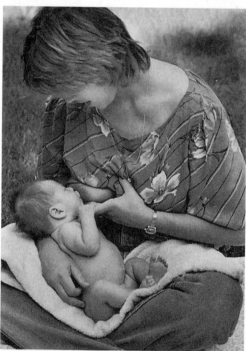

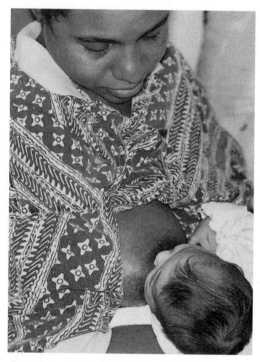

Once you are confident and breastfeeding is going well, then you can breastfeed anywhere and in a variety of positions that work well for you and your baby.

This position would be very difficult for a newborn. The baby, who is four weeks old, is well supported (with his head at the level of his mother's breast and his body resting on a folded towel on her lap) but his body is not facing his mother's, nor is it tucked in close, so he must turn his head towards his mother to feed.

This mother has turned her five-day-old baby's body toward hers and tucked her in close before starting to feed. The baby's head rests on her forearm (not in the crook of her elbow), and she supports her baby's lower back and bottom with her hand.

3. **Use props for support.** Have as many pillows, cushions, or soft, firm supports (such as folded rugs or blankets as well as whatever you may need to support your feet) as you need to support both you and your baby.

4. **Remember to have a glass of water** or other beverage within your reach so you can drink something while breastfeeding, if you are thirsty.

5. **While getting yourself ready,** you may need to put the baby down beside you or have someone else hold the baby until you are ready to have him brought to you.

Two important things to avoid:

- *Do not* be tempted to sit leaning back in bed, or in a chair that is designed for lounging, without proper support behind your back.

- *Do not* be tempted to start feeding until you are comfortable and ready.

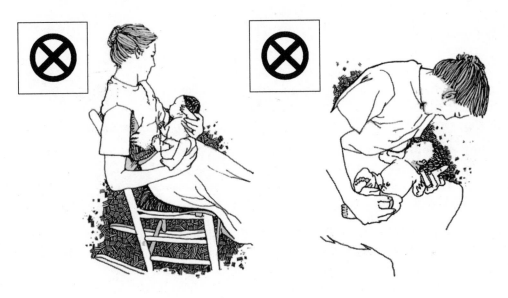

Once you and your baby have got breastfeeding right, you will get so used to feeding that you'll do it along with your ordinary activities—while you are on the phone, eating your dinner, or working at your desk. You'll have a spare hand for reading, cuddling your older child, or holding a cup. At the start though, learn what is most comfortable for you.

How You Hold Your Baby

Once you are comfortable, you need to hold your baby in a good position for her to be able to feed. *She needs to be comfortable, well supported, and not straining to get at your breast.*

You may find, at first, that it is easier for you to hold your baby with one arm or the other, depending whether you are right-handed or left-handed. With practice, it will get easier with the other arm.

If you have twins, practice feeding just one baby at a time at first. When you are good at it, you can try both at once.

- **Hold your baby tucked in very close to your body, with her body turned in towards yours.** She should not have to turn her head to reach your breast. Her front should be tucked in close to your body, secure but not tight.

There are no rules about which of your hands should be used for what. The important things are:

1. *Your baby should feel secure and supported.*

2. *She must have good, easy access to your breast.*

Look at the pictures in this section. Note how the women are holding their babies. Even though the babies are in similar positions close to their mothers, the women are holding them differently. *Work out what is best for you and your baby.*

- **Her whole body, especially from her head to her bottom, should be well supported.** Use your hands and your arms and possibly pillows too to support her if you are sitting up. If you are lying down, she will be lying on her side on the bed or floor, on pillows or on your arm.

- **She needs to be held so that her mouth will be at the same level as your nipple when she feeds.** She should not have to pull down or away from your breast once she is on your breast. This means that she should not be held above the level of your nipple. If anything, she should be held *just below* your nipple as you prepare to bring her to your breast.

- **Her head, neck, and back should be in almost a straight line.** Her head should not be tilted down. She will not be able to swallow in that position. If anything, her head should be tilted *slightly* backward so her chin presses into your breast.

Note: Good positioning for your baby never requires her to turn her head to take your breast when she is young. Whatever position you and she are in, cradle her close to you, with her mouth in front of and just below your nipple. Look carefully at the pictures in this book, and look at how well supported the babies are, and how close they are to their mothers' bodies.

A special tip on clothing. Wearing comfortable clothing helps in getting positioning right. If you have to fuss with tight or uncomfortable clothes, it will get in the way of you and your baby. Try to wear clothes that are comfortable and in which you can feed discreetly if you are outside your home. A big shawl or scarf can be useful here. A loose top that can be pulled up is often more discreet and comfortable than a blouse that buttons down the front.

Do you or your baby prefer one side or the other? Some babies prefer feeding from one breast rather than the other. Sometimes shifting the baby's position at the breast helps, holding the baby in an under-the-arm position, so that she approaches both breasts the same way. Sometimes nothing helps, and one breasts becomes larger than the other from having its milk always more stimulated than the other.

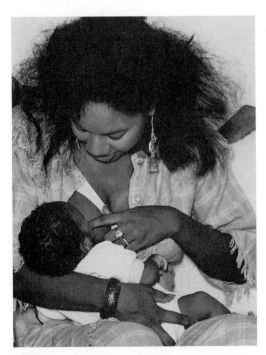

It is important that a young baby's body and head are in a straight line during feeding. The head must be at the level of the mother's breast, but the body can slope downward, as long as it does not cause the baby to pull down on the breast. This mother's fingers are resting on her breast—not applying pressure and pulling her breast away from the baby.

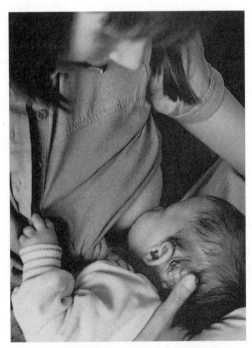

This is good positioning. Here a mother supports her baby's neck and shoulders in her hand, with her thumb and fingers resting on the back of his head. Notice how the baby's chin is neither tilted up nor dropped back.

In summary, the important points to remember about how you hold your baby are that your baby:

1. *Is held close to you*

2. *Is well supported*

3. *Is turned towards you*

4. *Has her mouth just below your nipple as you prepare to feed*

5. *Has her head, neck, and back all in a straight line*

6. *Make sure her arms and hands do not get in the way as she gets on to feed*

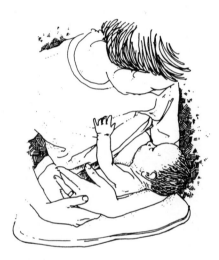 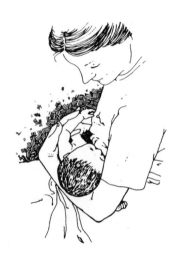

The important things to avoid are as follows:

1. Do *not* lie your baby on her back. She would have to turn her head to find your breast.

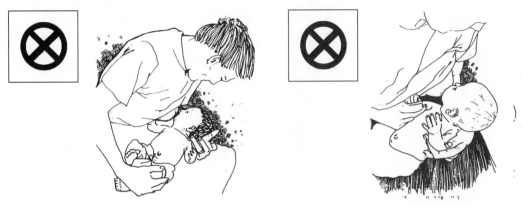

2. Do *not* hold her so that her mouth is above or well below your nipple.

3. Do *not* let her chin push down toward her chest.

4. Do *not* bring your breast to the baby, bring your baby to the breast.

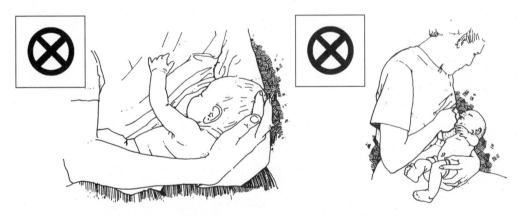

Some Important Information on Supporting Your Breast

Once you and your baby are confident with breastfeeding, you may not need to support your breast. But in the early days it can often help.

Breast support may be necessary only while you are putting your baby onto your breast. Once she is on and suckling, some women will find they can slowly take their hand away. But don't do this until you're sure the baby is on well.

You can use either hand, under either breast. Use whichever hand is not supporting your baby. Place your hand flat against your ribcage, with your thumb up

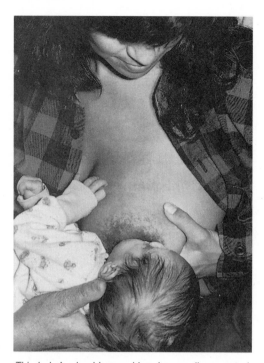

This baby's shoulders and head are well supported with the opposite hand, so the mother's other hand is free to support her breast. Note how she keeps her thumb well back from the areola and does not press it down on the breast.

and way back away from your areola. You may find it helpful if you use your index and middle finger to support the underside of your breast if it is large, and to push up on your breast from underneath if your breast is small. Doing this seems to make a great deal of difference in the first days, as it makes it easier for your baby to grasp your breast.

Remember, you are *supporting* it, not holding it tightly, and certainly not letting your fingers dig into your breast, which would be uncomfortable and change the shape. Just feel the weight of your breast rest on our fingers. Look carefully at the picture here of how to do this.

Your hand is simply supporting your breast to make it a bit firmer as your baby goes on, and to lift it slightly so your baby is not supporting its weight with his chin. It is not intended to squeeze your breast into a different shape; that will not help, and may pull the breast partly out of your baby's mouth. Be especially careful not to let your thumb press into your breast. You may be able to remove your hand once your baby is feeding well.

If you have small breasts, you may not need to support them at all.

If you have large breasts, you may need to support them throughout the whole feed.

The woman on page 49, who has large breasts, is using a band of soft material (a long stretch of broad bandage or a long woven belt would do) tied around her neck, looped under her breast. We've been told this has been a traditional practice among some North American Indians. It is tied tight enough to give good support to her breast, but not tight enough to distort the shape of the part of the breast and the nipple offered to her baby. It can be slipped off the first breast and looped under the second breast when necessary.

If you are out and about when feeding, then take this band with you. It would be best to wear a front-fastening blouse; just slip the band over your head and around your breast, and feed as normal.

Alternatively, use your hand under your breast throughout the feed, as the woman in this picture is doing. If you want to free up your hand, use your ingenuity—a small soft child's ball or stuffed animal, or even part of a cardboard tube from a kitchen roll will work well too!

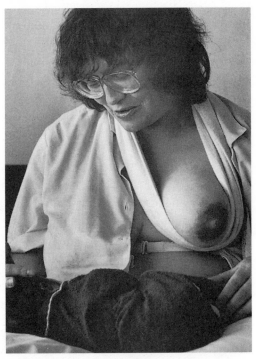

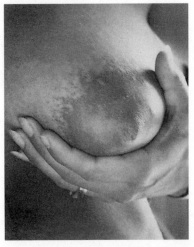

If you need to support your breast, place your fingers and palm of the hand underneath and rest your thumb lightly on top of the breast (but well back from the areola) or back toward your armpit. This way you are less likely to distort the shape of the breast as the baby feeds.

This woman has large, soft breasts. She is using a band of soft material (an elasticized fabric) around her neck and under her breast to give it support and better shape for the baby to suckle. This way both of her hands are free to support her newborn and help him take her breast.

How Your Baby Takes Your Breast

These principles of how your baby takes your breast are the same for all mothers and babies, even if you have inverted nipples or a small or sick baby. It will be more difficult if you have these problems. It will probably take longer and you will need lots of patience, but it can work! (See pages 91-92 if you have inverted nipples, and pages 98-102 if you have a small or sick baby.)

This part will work well only if you have arranged yourself and your baby comfortably and well. If you and he are comfortably together, then you will be able to carry out these steps to encourage him to take your breast.

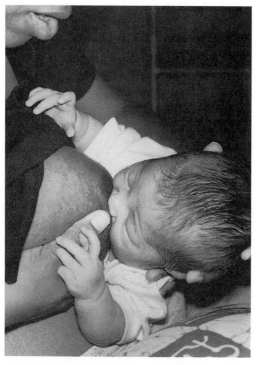

This mother is sitting upright and using the opposite arm to hold her baby so that her baby's nose is at the level of her nipple.

Notice how she gently cradles the baby's head with her fingers, which gives her just enough control to make sure the baby is well on the breast. By resting this arm on a pillow she avoids strain to her back and shoulders.

- **Support your baby well** across his shoulder and the base of his head. You can do this in either of two ways:

  a. Cradle him on the inside of your forearm, on the same side on which he is feeding. You will support his shoulder and neck on your arm just below your elbow.

  b. Support him with the arm on the opposite side from the breast he is feeding from. Cradle his shoulders, his neck, and the base of his head lightly on your hand. This is for support only. Do not put pressure on his head. His back should rest on the inside of your forearm.

- **Hold his head gently.**

- **Brush your baby's lips lightly against your nipple,** to give him a sense of what to take in his mouth. This is how he knows the breast is there. If he is well positioned, he should be right by your nipple.

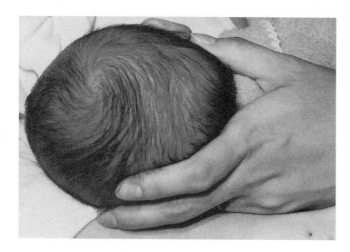

A newborn baby's head is very sensitive and needs to be held gently, especially if the baby has had a difficult passage at birth.

This mother places the palm of her hand on her baby's upper back and shoulders, leaving her fingers free to bring the baby on to her breast.

- **Wait until his mouth is wide open before letting him take your breast in his mouth.** He has a reflex to do this; you simply need to encourage this reflex.

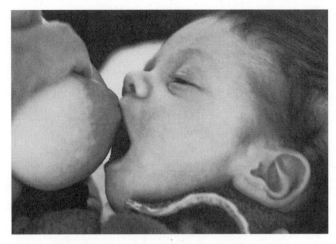

Look at this baby's wide gape and how his nostrils are at the level of the nipple. This is the correct position for the baby going on the breast, since it is actually the baby's lower jaw, pressed against the breast, that does the work.

When his mouth is opening wide, quickly but gently move him onto your breast so he can take a good, deep mouthful. (This may take practice to get the timing right. If you wait too long, he will have begun to close his mouth by the time you bring him onto the breast.)

You may have to work with this for a few minutes before he gapes his mouth open widely enough to take in enough of your breast. Don't worry about this. Some babies are sleepy. Some are not too hungry. *All babies have to learn to feed well.* Calmly repeat the action of lightly brushing his lips against your nipple until he responds by opening his mouth wide.

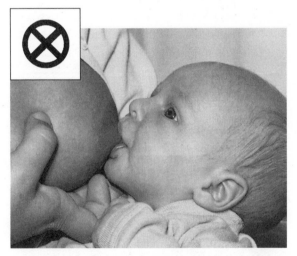

This baby is not well on the breast. He is nipple feeding. If he were allowed to continue to do this, his mother could become very sore. The baby may not grow well, or may have colic.

If he or you become frustrated or cry, then stop. Breathe slowly. Calm yourself. Calm him. Try again. Start slowly. It does not matter if feeding takes a long time in the early days; you will both become better as your practice. If you are both crying or if you are tense, it helps to have someone else calm the baby and calm you. Ask for a back rub or neck massage or cup of tea or whatever will make you feel better.

- **Make sure he takes a large mouthful of your breast, not just your nipple.**
  To do this, he needs to use his whole bottom jaw and tongue. Think about where the baby's bottom lip, rather than his top lip, make contact with your breast. (It is his lower jaw that does the work in extracting the milk.) Your nipple will then end up right at the back of his mouth, where it cannot be damaged by suction or friction.

  Look at the diagram and photograph on pages 56 and 57 to see where your nipple should be. Look too at how your baby's tongue should lie right over his gum, covering it. In this position his tongue and bottom jaw will move rhythmically up and down against your breast to get the milk. His tongue will lie over his bottom gum throughout the feed; it will not move in and out. In fact, you (or someone guiding you) may see his tongue if you just tip back the edge of his lower lip while he is feeding well (but be careful not to disturb him if you do this).

  This photograph (below) of the baby with her tongue on her lower gum shows you where the tongue is when feeding well.

  The mouthful of breast that your baby takes in should be all the way around and behind your nipple, and include some of the dark area around your nipple (the areola). Some women with small areolas find that the baby takes it all in; some women with large areolas can see quite a lot of it.

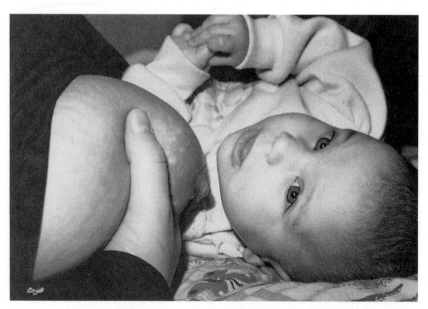

This baby has just come off the breast. You can still see her tongue, which is thrust forward during breastfeeding and completely covers her low gum.

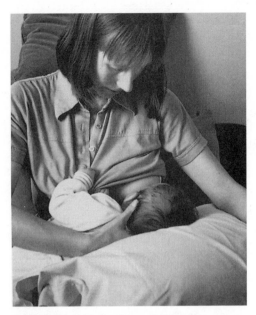

Once your baby is feeding well, there is nothing else you need to do. You can relax and enjoy it.

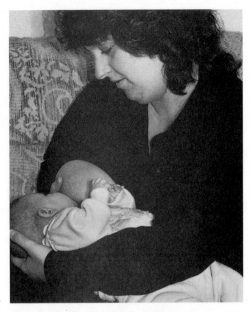

This three-month-old baby is well supported, with a hand behind her shoulders and fingers cradling her head. Her body rests on her mother's lap.

If this were a young infant, then her body would need to be turned on its side and tucked in close. This detail is not so important for an older infant, who can easily turn from the waist.

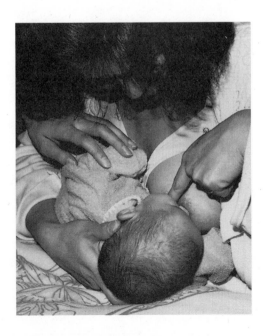

Sometimes you need to take the baby off your breast, because she is not attached well and is causing you pain. Here the mother is learning how to break suction gently. The helper is gently holding the baby's arm so that the mother can see what she is doing. Place your finger in the corner of her mouth (many mothers use their little finger), press down on your breast tissue (which breaks the suction), and draw your nipple out as you take her off.

If you can still see some areola, more of it should show beyond your baby's top lip than beyond his bottom lip. *It will be hard for you to see this, because it is difficult to see looking down on yourself.*

You cannot easily see under your own breast. You can ask a helper what your baby and breast look like when he is feeding, or sit beside a mirror to see for yourself. The picture on page 55 shows what it should look like.

Remember that breastfed babies *take* the breast; it is not like bottle feeding, where babies are *given* the bottle teat.

(In some countries, such as the United States, the word nipple is used for the rubber or plastic tip of the bottle on which the baby sucks. In this book we use the word *nipple* only to describe the nipple on a woman's breast; this is sensitive, stretchy, and responsive. Rubber or plastic objects are not. We use the word *teat* throughout this book to describe the rubber or plastic tip of the bottle.)

- **Relax and let the feed happen.** If for any reason you feel your baby is not well positioned, especially if it is painful for you, stop the feed. Take him off the breast gently by breaking the suction; you can do this by slipping a finger in his mouth. (It is best to do this with short fingernails.) Take a few slow breaths to calm yourself. Then calm him and start again.

What to Do if Breastfeeding Hurts

Breastfeeding should not hurt, other than perhaps a brief pain during the first few sucks of each feed, in the first few days (or for the first day or two after you have begun working on a problem). *If it hurts, then usually the positioning is not right. Stop feeding, take your baby off your breast. Take a few calming breaths and try again.*

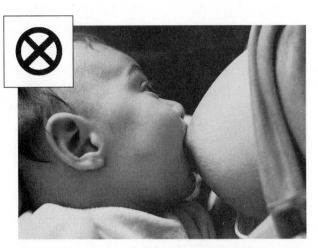

Because nipple pain and damage is usually caused by positioning problems, there is no need to use any of the over-the-counter or pre-scription creams, sprays, or lotions that may be recommended to you, or that you seen in drug or chemist shops. These can actually cause nipple damage by interfering with the normal balance of organisms on the skin. Nor do you need to prepare your nipples in pregnancy (by using methods that supposedly toughen and prevent them from getting sore or cracked), or prepare them by washing them before you feed. If the positioning is right, then nothing else is needed. You or a helper can look for these signs to see if your baby is feeding well.

This baby is not well positioned. Can you see how this positioning may not permit the baby to get enough milk (and therefore not stimulate enough milk to be produced for the next feed) and would be likely to result in sore nipples or worse?

Note how she seems to be pulling down and off the breast. There is also a gap between her chin and the breast and her nose is not resting against the breast.

1. Your baby should have gaped his mouth widely enough and be tucked in close enough that he should have taken a large mouthful of breast.

2. Your baby's lower lip should be

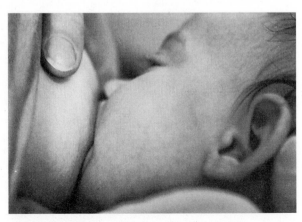

Here this same baby is positioned just right on the opposite breast. She is now tucked in close, her mouth open wide, and her chin. She has taken in a good mouthful and is feeding well.

in contact with the breast, not pinching in at the base of the nipple.

3. His nose should not be touching your breast; if it does he is not well positioned. *There should be no need for you to hold your breast away from his nose to let him breathe.* You should see his top lip pressed against the breast and there should be a small gap between top lip and the splayed nostrils. Tuck his body in closer to you, if necessary, to widen the gap a little between his nose and your breast.

4. His bottom lip should be turned back against your breast, and his bottom jaw should be firmly pressing into the underside of your breast.

    This is hard for you to see, but you should be able to feel the sensation from the tip of the tongue and the jaw moving together at a point that is well onto your breast, *not* up close to your nipple.

    Do not try to look at this part in too much detail, as moving your baby or your breast to have a look will disturb your baby. Instead, shut your eyes and feel the sensation of his tongue and jaws. Remember that it should not hurt at all.

5. Your baby will take a few quick sucks, and then start to suck strongly, deeply, and rhythmically. You will notice that he will have a pattern of sucking a few times and then pausing, sucking again a few times, and then pausing again.

    He will do this throughout the feed. He will vary the strength of his sucks every now and then, but mostly they should be regular, deep, and strong.

    As the feed goes on, he will pause for longer periods, and the bouts of sucking will get shorter. Do not be tempted to take him off the breast at this point. He needs to continue feeding. This is explained on page 71.

6. Your baby will continue to feed peacefully and well until he decides he has had enough. At that time he will let go of your breast. *There is no need for you to take him off. He will show you that he has had enough when that time comes.*

7. Feeding should not hurt you. People mistakenly think that pain is a normal part of breastfeeding. It is not. You may feel an unusual sensation as his sucking stretches your nipple. Some women even feel a quick stab of pain around the nipple just as the baby starts, which passes in a few seconds. This will last only for the first few days.

    One sensation you may feel is a strong tingling, like a mild electrical charge, as you release your milk (see page 69). This too is normal, although not something women usually feel in the early days or weeks. It is also normal not to feel anything tingling at all; some women do, some don't.
    Special tip: Occasionally some babies who are feeding well come off the breast

for a few seconds, not long after they have started to feed. Then they soon go back on again. These babies show no signs of distress and there is no pain for the mothers. We believe that these babies need to come off briefly, either because the milk flow is too fast to cope with, or because they need to burp or pass wind.

Once your baby has taken the first side well, he will want a short rest. He may or may not decide to take the second side (see page 71).

After your baby is finished with one breast, it is a good moment to change his diaper or nappy if necessary. You can then see if he is interested in taking the second side. *Give him the choice.* He may be finished.

The same principles of positioning apply to the second side. Be just as careful, let him come off the breast himself when he has finished.

Some babies cry immediately after a good feed. Hunger can be eliminated as a cause. See pages 130-134 for what to do if this happens.

In summary, *what is important about how your baby takes your breast is that at*

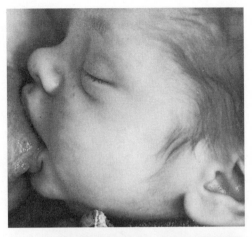

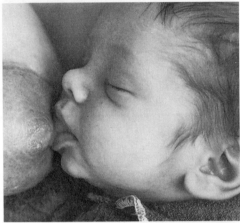

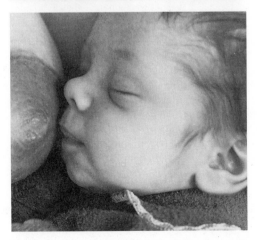

In this series you can see how the baby comes off the breast by herself when she has had enough.

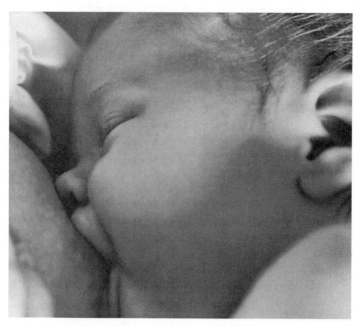

When breastfeeding is going well, the mother's nipple is never damaged because it is so far back into the baby's mouth there is no friction against it. (It is friction that causes both soreness and damage to the nipple.) This is why breastfeeding should not hurt.

In this photograph, and the accompanying drawing and diagram, you can see what is going on inside your baby's mouth when breastfeeding is going well.

Notice that when the baby is well on the breast her lower lip is pressed down flat against her chin and she has taken not only the nipple but also a large amount of breast tissue into her mouth, forming them into a teat with her tongue.

The baby's nose is against the breast but not pressing in. You can see how the nostrils in this drawing flare to the side, which makes it possible for her nose to be right against your breast and for her still to be able to breathe. Look at your baby and see how her nostrils are designed so that she can breathe comfortably while breastfeeding.

In the diagram, see how your baby's tongue should completely cover her lower gum (or teeth) and protect your nipple, which lies safely in the back of the baby's mouth where it cannot be damaged.

You can see very little of this mother's large areola, because most of it is in the baby's mouth. Look at how the nipple plus breast tissue together are pulled into the shape of a teat.

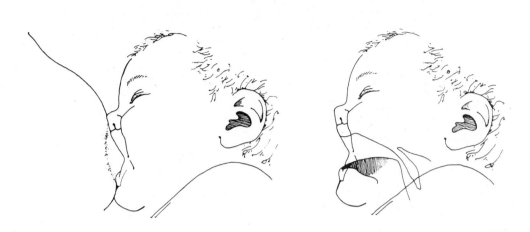

KEY:

1. nipple
2. areola and breast tissue, with underlying milk ducts
3. baby's tongue
4. breast
5. baby's throat

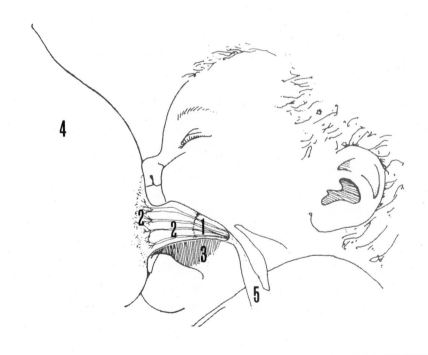

each feed your baby should:

1. *Gape his mouth widely.*

2. *Take a large mouthful of breast.*

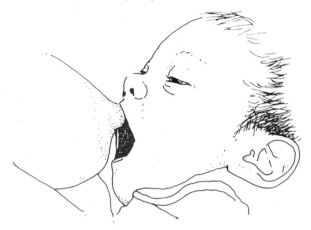

3. *Such mostly strongly and rhythmically, with pauses between each episode of*

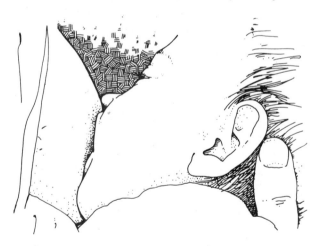

sucking.

4. *Have no problem breathing.*

5. *Easily bring up any air bubbles (burp/wind) if you sit him up. Remember to sup-*

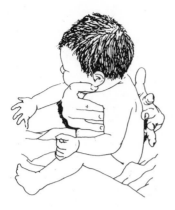

port his head.

6. *Come off the breast himself when he has finished.*

Remember that feeding should not hurt you at all.

The important things to avoid are as follows:

- Do *not* try to put your breast into your baby's mouth. Simply help him take it by moving him to your breast.

- Do *not* let him feed if it hurts you; take him off and try again.

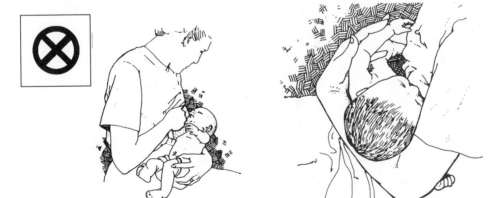

- Do *not* let him continue to feed if he sucks rapidly and lightly *all the time*. Take him off and try again.

- Do *not* continue to feed if he seems distressed. Calm yourself, calm him, and try again.

One Mother's Experience of Learning to Breastfeed Well:
The First Two Weeks

With my first child, Colin, I had sore, cracked nipples, and breastfeeding didn't become pleasant for six weeks. That's how long it took for me to learn how to put him on my breast right and for him to know what to do. I didn't realize he was sucking on my nipple and that's why I was sore. Once he was on my breast, I let him stay for half an hour or more or until he fell asleep because he would scream if I took him off. Colin never came off the breast on his own. Sometimes I would hardly get a break between feeds.

Finally I found a breastfeeding support group listed in the phone directory. I called, told them about my symptoms, and asked for help. I was able to heal my nipples, even the cracked one, by letting them air after each feed until they were completely dry and by teaching Colin to take much more of the breast in his mouth. For a while I had to pay close attention each time I put him on or he would not get it right. Once we learned to breastfeed correctly, everything was fine. He didn't wean fully until eighteen months, and by that time he was only taking my breast for a few minutes several times a day, for comfort.

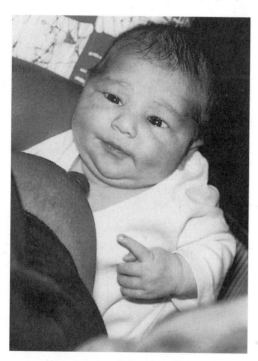

Here, two-day-old Devi is still learning how to take her mother's breast, which is already quite large and firm and has a large nipple that does not stand erect. Like her brother before her, Devi has a small mouth compared to the size of her mother's nipple and breast.

I have big nipples, and both my babies have had small mouths. Colin was born with the habit of sucking his bottom lip and not opening his mouth very wide to feed. I had to teach him how to take my breast. And I have had to do the same with Devi, my daughter.

Devi sucked strongly from the first feed, and she has always opened her mouth wide. She seemed to take my breast well until my milk came in fully at forty-eight hours. I think my breast was really stimulated to produce because she sucked so strongly. I suddenly became very full and that, combined with the size of my nipples and the fact that they didn't stand erect, prevented her from getting my breast into her mouth. She began to scream at each feed, to shake her head when I put her on, to spit out the nipple and to refuse the breast. It was a struggle for a few days.

I began to apply warmth to my breasts between feeds, using a heating pad or standing under a warm shower. This made me feel more comfortable, took down some of the swelling, and softened by breast tissue, making it easier for Devi to take my breast. My husband bought a hand pump for me, and I expressed as much milk as I felt comfortable with before each feed. I would drop some milk directly into her mouth when it was open from crying, and as soon as she'd tasted it, I'd put her on while she was still crying and her mouth was open. She would suck two or three times, get upset, pull off, and start crying again. The third and fourth days after her birth were the hardest. I was very upset, and I was afraid of repeating what had happened with Colin.

I tried to keep myself calm, but it was hard for those two days. She seemed so hungry and yet so upset (as upset as I was). Once during the night, my husband gave her a bottle of my expressed milk, and the next afternoon I fed her another bottle to make sure she would not lose weight. Then I called my midwife, who stayed on the phone, talking me through a whole feed. Then she suggested I send my husband to get me a beer so I would relax—that helped too.

My husband is very helpful. He is taking off almost a month of vacation time and unpaid leave from his job to be home with us, to take care of Colin, who is twenty-three months, and to run the house. During the hardest days he gave me back rubs whenever I wanted, even in the middle of the night.

For the entire first week we kept the answering machine on, and I talked on the phone only a little each day, and never when I was feeding Devi. Colin is very active and our house is very small, a three-

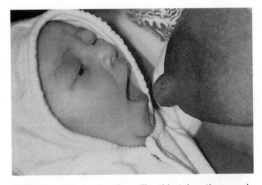

Breastfeeding in situations like this takes time, and practice, and a great deal of patience in the first days, as both mother and baby must learn to get it right.

Lawan first had to teach Devi to open her mouth wide before she could have the breast. This was frustrating for Devi for several days, until she learned.

A few babies can be put on the breast when they are crying, while their mouth is open wide. But, as with most babies, this did not work for Devi. She would cry so hard that she didn't notice when the breast was in her mouth. So Lawan first had to calm her and then coax her to open her mouth. Dripping a little breast milk into her mouth when she first began to cry helped.

room cottage with a tiny garden, but we tried to keep it quiet and played soft music. That helped all of us. We also tried to keep visitors to a minimum. We put a sign on our door and told our friends and relatives who dropped by or called that we would love for them to bring us meals but that we probably couldn't spend time with them. Most days someone has brought food, and that has been wonderful, allowing us to spend time with Colin and Devi.

By the time Devi was thirteen days, I had finally taught her to take my breast well. For a few days, each time I breastfed I encouraged her by talking to her and gently rocking her. I had learned to hold her whole body very close to me and to keep her wrapped because she prefers being swaddled to having her arms and legs free. I had to feed in a sitting position, making sure my back was straight up and down, to make it work. Feeding times got easier and better each day. She fed well once on the breast and came off on her own when she was done. She'd look at me much of the time she fed. We were really lucky; she already slept five hours at a stretch at night.

Devi cried at the breast and fought feeding only in the middle of the night. I think she was very hungry then and became frustrated more easily. She sometimes took ten or fifteen minutes to get going at that feed; but I didn't give her any choice but to take my breast and eventually she did! At that point I hadn't needed to express milk in three days; my nipples weren't cracked; and if Devi

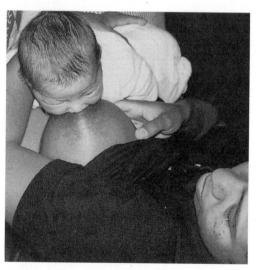

Here, ten days after birth, Devi is feeding well. Lawan still has to be careful at each feed, making sure both she and Devi are in good, comfortable positions and that Devi's head is at the level of her breast and her nose at the level of Lawan's nipple before Lawan puts her on.

didn't go on correctly and sucked on the nipple, I immediately took her off and tried again. Even when everything was right. there was some mild soreness during her first few sucks; but after that there was no pain or soreness. I was beginning to enjoy it!

For the first three weeks I could only breastfeed sitting upright. After that, Devi learned to feed while I was lying on my side, as long as she was not too hungry. When she was four weeks I could nurse sitting or lying anywhere. When Devi was five weeks I began expressing milk regularly so that my husband could give her a bottle of breastmilk each day, which allowed me to have some free time. I find this especially helpful if we are in the car and she gets hungry.

Devi is now six weeks and knows how to go on the breast. She feeds well and sleeps five or six hours at a stretch each night. She's an alert, peaceful baby. Breastfeeding is great.

In this photograph (page 64) you can see a bit of Devi's right arm, which Lawan has been careful to place underneath her breast so that it does not get in the way and prevent her from tucking Devi in close to her body. Lawan has a pillow supporting her own forearm, upon which Devi's head rests. She uses another pillow to support Devi's lower body.

A Note for Helpers

If you are helping a mother to breastfeed, then take time to think about your own position.

You should be comfortable, so that you can take all the time that you need, without getting uncomfortable or tired.

You will find the positions that suit you best. Two suggested positions are:

- Sitting beside the mother, side by side, facing the same direction (see picture). You should sit on the side opposite the breast the mother is feeding from (unless the mother is holding the baby under her arm), on a chair at the same height as her.

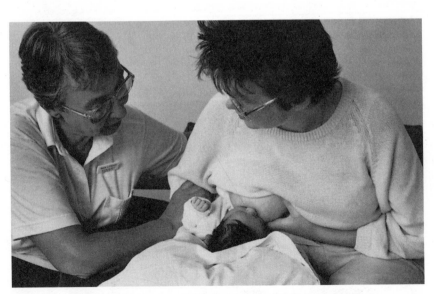

If you are helping a mother with breastfeeding, be sure to sit down close to her. Make sure that your back is comfortable and that you don't have to strain to reach over and assist her.

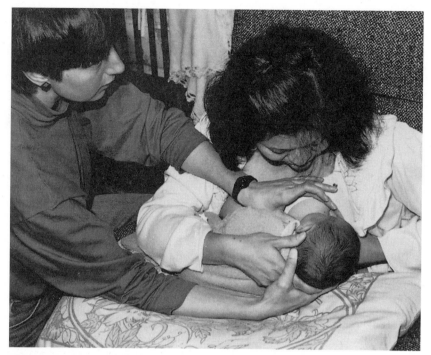

If a mother needs hands-on guidance, place your hands ON TOP of hers so that she can feel how to do it herself. Then watch her do it herself and give her feedback.

- Sitting beside the mother, facing in the opposite direction. Again, you should be on the opposite side from the breast the mother is feeding from, and at the same height as her.

Work with the mother to guide her, rather than doing it for her. She does not need a helper who will only put her baby on her breast and then leave her. The best care is when you suggest to the mother what she can do, and then watch and guide her in getting it right, or put your hands over hers and let her feel what you are doing. Remember to be patient and reassuring; the most important thing you can give a mother is confidence. A calm, positive manner is as important as skill in positioning the baby.

The picture here shows you how you can guide the mother's hands.

For mothers and helpers: It is essential when a mother needs help, the helper has easy access to both her and her breasts. In most countries, this is considered quite normal. In the United States some helpers do not work in this way; for fear of legal action, they do not touch women's breasts. It is unhelpful and unproductive to try to work with a woman while avoiding touching her breasts. Some women need skilled hands-on care. If you are one of these women, persist in finding someone who will work directly with you, your baby, and your breasts. Or look in the resource section of this book for organizations that may help.

If all else fails, work with a close friend or family member, using this book to guide you.

About Milk Supply and Milk Release

While you and your baby are working to get breastfeeding right, your body is also working to get the milk supply and composition right.

Milk Supply

Just as in pregnancy your hormones changed to support a growing baby, so after birth your hormones change to make milk.

Your breasts have already been prepared by the pregnancy hormones, and they are already making the essential early milk, or colostrum, for your baby. These hormones also limit the amount made to the small volume your new baby needs at first. As soon as your baby is born, the milk-producing hormone, prolactin, starts to work on your breasts to make a generous milk supply.

Your breasts respond to your baby feeding. As your baby feeds, your brain reads the message that your breasts need to make more milk to replace what your baby is taking. It therefore releases prolactin, which gives the signal to your breasts to make more milk. The milk taken from your breasts is simply replaced. In this way there is always enough—and usually more than your baby needs.

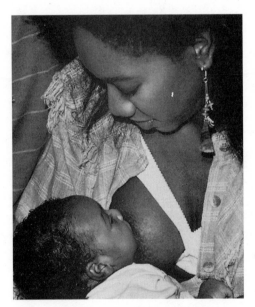

As your baby feeds, your body responds by making more milk to replace what your baby has taken.

If your baby does not feed well, then the message your breasts will get after a while is that the baby doesn't need much milk, so they will not produce as much.

Understanding this helps you to work out:

1. How a good milk supply builds up

2. How to treat milk supply problems if they occur

3. How to build up a good milk supply even if your baby is small or sick and you cannot feed her directly.

Make sure that your baby always feeds well, especially in the early days and weeks as your supply becomes established. Limiting your baby's time on the breast, or not getting

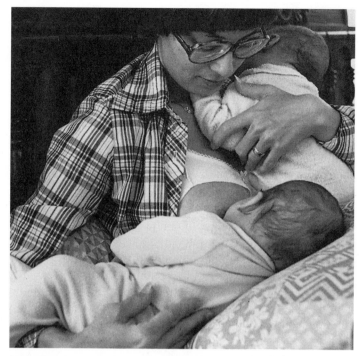

You can produce plenty of milk to feed twins—even triplets. But in the early days it is easier to feed one baby at a time, even though this takes a lot longer. When you become more confident and your babies know how to take the breast, then you can try feeding both babies at once.

her well positioned (so that she doesn't get enough milk) will result in your breasts not getting the message to make enough milk.

This balance between the amount your baby needs and the amount your breasts make is so finely tuned that if you have twins, your body will make enough milk for two. All you need to do is help both babies to breastfeed well. Some women have even breastfed triplets (though this is difficult, and you need lots of help).

If you cannot feed your baby for a time, then make sure your breasts still get the right signal to make milk by removing the milk that is there. If she is in a special care or intensive care unit, if you are so ill you cannot breastfeed, or if you are separated for any reason, then express your milk regularly (see pages 86-90); or ask for help if you are ill. This is especially important in the first week or two after birth. Do not worry if you do not have much of a supply. You can build up your supply when you and the baby are home.

Milk Release

After producing milk, your breasts need to release it. Milk comes out as a result of a combination of

1. The letdown reflex and

2. Your baby feeding well

When you feed your baby, or sometimes even if you just think about your baby or hear her cry, your breasts will let down the milk. This means that the small muscles around the areas where milk is stored in your breast contract and squeeze the milk out.

Some women will feel this letdown like a tingle in their breasts, and others will not feel it at all. Some women find that they feel it more as the baby gets bigger. The surest sign that it is happening is contented swallowing by the baby.

Oxytocin is the hormone responsible for sending the letdown signal to your breasts. This is the same hormone that was responsible for your labor contractions. It is also released when you make love.

You may find that in the early days, your womb contracts whenever you breastfeed. This is oxytocin at work. You will lose more blood around the time of feeding as a result of these contractions, which helps to clear your uterus of the blood and other substances it needs to lose.

With breastfeeding, your womb will also contract down to size more quickly, but it may be painful as it does this. Some women find that these afterbirth contractions, or afterpains, become more painful the more children they have. The feeling will last for only a day or two.

Because oxytocin is also released when you make love, you may find that you release milk at that time. This is normal, but it is useful to have a towel handy so as to avoid a damp bed. It can also help if you feed your baby before making love, to minimize milk release and untimely interruptions by the baby. Because oxytocin is released during both lovemaking and breastfeeding, some find that breastfeeding makes them feel sexy. This is quite normal; enjoy it while it lasts.

Sometimes milk is released at times when you do not expect it. Thinking about your baby when you are away from her, or hearing another baby cry can cause milk to let down.

Sometimes women find it hard to release their milk in stressful situations. Oxytocin is not released and the milk flow will be delayed. For this to happen, however, the stress has to be fairly severe; just feeling a bit anxious is most unlikely to do it. And it is very rare for this to happen in the early weeks after birth.

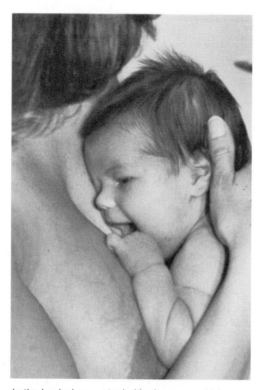

In the beginning, oxytocin (the hormone which causes milk to come down) is released in your body when your baby feeds. As your baby gets older, oxytocin can also be released when you are feeling warm and close, when you hear her cry, or when you think she might be ready for a feed (even if you are not anywhere near her!).

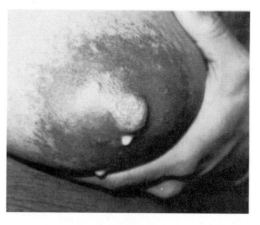

Your milk may sometimes drip from your breast when your baby is not feeding. This is the result of the letdown reflex. But don't worry if this does not happen—some women breastfeed very well without ever seeing this.

You can often solve a milk release problem by getting your baby to feed right. For example, if your baby has not been well positioned, your nipples may be sore and you may be tense and anxious, especially if your baby is crying. Then oxytocin might not be released. Getting your baby into a correct position (remember, this includes getting yourself into a comfortable position too) so that you can feed well even once will almost always break the cycle of tension and anxiety that interferes with letdown. Work on positioning for both you and your baby, and ask for help if it is available. As soon as she is feeding well, your nipples will not be sore, you will feel better, and her strong, rhythmic feeding will cause your letdown. Then you will relax.

Sometimes people suggest that the main problem is that you are tense. Of course you will be anxious if you cannot get your baby to feed. The solution to a letdown problem might not be simply to try to relax; it is possible that the more you "try to relax" the more tense you will become. Some women find that gentle nipple stimulation or placing a warm wet cloth on the breast helps cause a letdown. Others say that visualizing helps; trying imagining a waterfall or standing in a lovely shower of water. See what works best for your body.

It is often the case that having one good feed solves what had been a serious problem. This happens because

- Your baby is no longer crying from hunger and frustration.

- She has learned to do it right once, so it is easier the next time.

- You have learned to do it right once, and will be more skilled the next time.

- You feel more confident.

Milk and Milk Composition

Breast milk is a constantly changing food that adjusts to the age and needs of your baby.

The composition of your breast milk is never constant. The amount of protein, fat, sugar (lactose), and other components change. The milk you produce if your baby is delivered prematurely is different from milk you would produce after nine months of pregnancy. And that milk is different from the milk you will produce after a few months. Mothers make milk that is suited to the needs of their own babies.

The first milk your body produces is called *colostrum*. This looks yellowish and creamy. A small amount of it is produced, but it is exactly what is needed, and you should not need to supplement with anything else. Colostrum is high in protein and helps your baby resist infection. It also acts as a laxative, helping babies pass the thick, green/black meconium (the first stool). This is important in reducing the risk of development of jaundice (see pages 136-138).

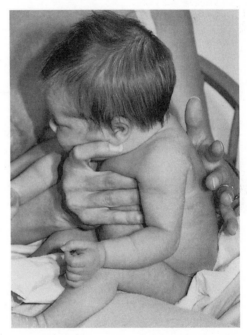

A breastfed baby is very easy to burp.

After your baby has finished one side, or if it seems like he needs to bring up a bubble in the middle of feeding on one side, sit him up so he can burp/wind. Support his chest and chin and gently rub his back. This should be all it takes to help him. Then offer him the breast once more.

In the first two or three days, your milk will gradually change from colostrum to mature breast milk. This milk is thinner and sometimes slightly bluish in color, rather than the yellow color of colostrum. Some women because anxious that their milk is not thick enough now to satisfy their babies. But in fact, it is all your baby needs for the next six months; normally, no artificial formula, water, or juice are needed.

Your body does all of this work for you, and you do not have to think about it or decide what your baby needs. But it is important to understand that the way in which you feed your baby can affect the composition of the milk that your baby takes.

Getting the Balance Right

Milk composition also changes throughout every breastfeed. The milk your baby takes at the end of a feed is different from the milk at the beginning of a feed. As you start she will get a lot of milk quickly. This milk (called the foremilk) is *high in volume, low in fat*. So although your baby gets a lot quickly, this milk is low in calories, but high in protein and other good things to help her grow and resist infection.

As your baby feeds, the composition of your milk gradually changes. After the first few minutes the *amount* of milk she gets slows down. You will see that her sucking also slows down, with longer pauses between periods of sucking.

As she sucks less frequently, she starts to get milk that is low in *quantity and higher in calories;* it is called the hindmilk. This is a gradual change that happens throughout the feed. It is not related to the timing of the letdown.

 It is essential that your baby get a good balance of both the foremilk and the hindmilk. Only in this way will she be able to take in enough milk and enough calories.

The only person who knows when your baby has had the right balance of foremilk and hindmilk is your baby.

Your baby understands her own appetite, and she knows when she is full. To ensure that she gets a good balance, therefore, all you need to do is:

- Let her feed when she is hungry.

- Let her stay on each breast until she has had enough and comes off herself.

The key to getting the balance right is to *let your baby finish the first breast first*. Then offer her the second side.

When she comes off the first side, sit her up. Let her burp if she needs to. (This is usually easy for breastfed babies.) Then offer her the second side. She will often take the second breast, but sometimes she will have had enough with one.

Problems that might occur in getting the balance right:

- Not positioning your baby well at your breast will result in her often not feeding long enough to get to the hindmilk.

- Limiting feeding time could cause problems for babies. Stopping her from feeding as often as she needs, or taking her off the breast after a set period of time might result in her not getting enough milk or enough calories.

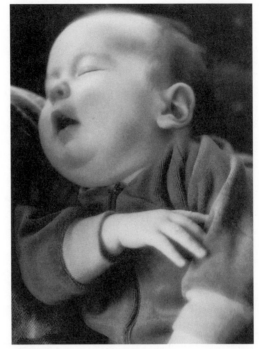

Sometimes it is very easy to tell when your baby has had enough.

Don't Impose Rules

There are no rules about the amount of time babies need to stay at the breast.

Some babies take all they need in four or five minutes; others need forty to fifty minutes. This changes over time with each baby too; they may take longer when very young than when they are older. And there are times when they increase their feeding time over a day or two in order to boost milk production. Like adults, who sometimes eat a small meal and sometimes a three course dinner, your baby will sometimes feed for a short time, sometimes longer. Don't look at the clock to decide if she has had enough; look at your baby. Women breastfed thousands of years before clocks were invented.

Don't worry about trying to balance the foremilk and the hindmilk yourself. Your baby will tell you all you need to know. The important thing is that you do not interfere with the balance by limiting the frequency or length of feeds.

A tip: Sometimes you will need to interrupt a feed before your baby is finished. For example, you may need to answer the phone or get to the shops before they close. This is not a problem so long as you do not do it regularly. Every now and then. *It is essential to keep your life as normal as possible.*

Here is a summary of what is important about milk and milk composition:

- Let your baby take a good balance of quantity and quality (foremilk and hind-milk). to do this, *do not limit the number of times you feed or the length of each feed.*

- Let your baby *finish the first breast first.* Then offer her the second side to see if she wants to take more.

Things to avoid:

- Do *not* give a fixed, small number of feeds in a day.

- Do *not* take your baby off either the first or second breast before she is finished.

- Do *not* let your baby feed if she is not well positioned.

Making Sure You've Got it Right: A Checklist

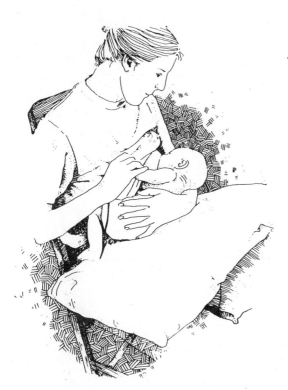

This list is a quick check over all the things you need to think about. You can find details in the previous sections if you need them.

1. Your own posture
(for details see pages 35-41)

You can feed in many different positions, and you should choose the ones that suit you.

First, make yourself comfortable.
This woman is seated in a straight-backed chair, with a cushion behind her shoulders and upper back to keep her upright. It may be easiest for you in the beginning to sit in a simple, straight-backed chair.

Here she sits in a deep couch. She has had to place several firm pillows behind her lower and upper back to bring her to a supported upright position. Although one leg is crossed over the other, she does have one foot flat on the floor. If her legs did not reach the floor, then she would need to put a book or cushion or box of the right height under her feet. On the other hand, if the sofa was too low and her thighs tilted upward, she would need to sit on an extra cushion. Her lap should be nearly flat.

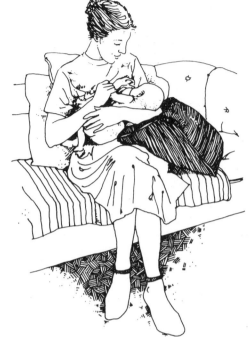

What do you see wrong in this picture about the woman's posture?

She is slouched and leaning to one side. If she does this for long her back muscles will get quite tense.

    She is also leaning back. If she feeds like this, her baby will have difficulty taking enough breast in his mouth and her breast will tend to pull out of his mouth as he feeds.

What does this woman need to do differently?

She needs to sit up straight in the chair, with her feet flat on the floor or on support of some other kind.

    She needs to move her bottom back in the chair so that the small of her back and her mid and upper back are fully supported.

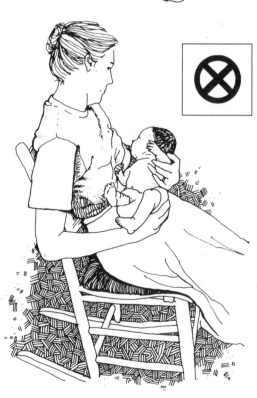

What do you see wrong in this picture about the woman's posture?

She is hunched over her baby and her shoulders look tense. If she does this for long, she will have an aching back.

What does this woman need to do differently?

She needs to sit up straight and let her shoulders relax. It will help if she has firm support behind her back, and a cushion to bring the baby just below her breast.

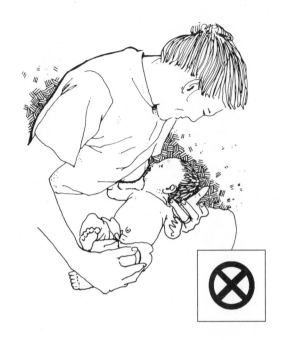

2. Holding your baby
(for details see pages 43-46)

Whatever body position you choose, you should hold your baby:

- Close to you
- In a way that is well supported
- With his body and head facing you
- With his mouth just below your nipple as you prepare to feed
- With his head, neck, and back in a straight line

Remember, the time you take to prepare—getting yourself and your baby in good positions—can prevent problems and even solve them if they occur.

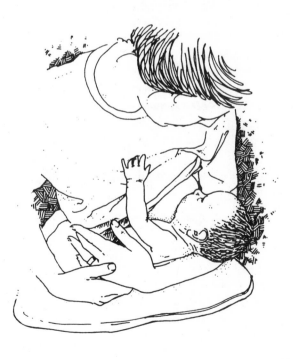

This woman has put a bed pillow on her lap to support her baby and also raise him to the level of her breast. Notice that the baby's body and head are in a straight line. This is also important.

Here, with both mother and baby lying on their sides, it is very easy for the mother to tuck the baby in close to her body and have the baby's head at the level of her breast.

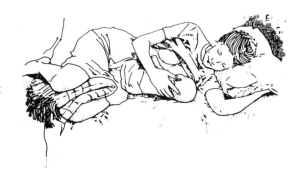

You will find this easiest to do if you start with your baby slightly lower than your breast before he goes on—with his nose level with your nipple when his mouth is closed.

The woman here is going to feed from her lower breast. A small pillow under her ribs may help to make this easier. If she feeds from the upper breast, then she will need to raise the baby up to the level of her breast with a cushion. Both her arms are then free to guide the baby to her breast.

Here is what it will look like from the side if you are feeding him while sitting up. Notice how his bottom hand is underneath his mother's breast and arm, out of the way. Here the baby's head rests on her forearm because she is holding him with the arm on the same side as the breast. If you use this arm, be sure he is on your forearm, NOT in the crook of your arm. We emphasize this point because bottle feeding has resulted in many women resting their baby's head in the crook of their arm. This results in the baby having to pull the breast to the side to feed.

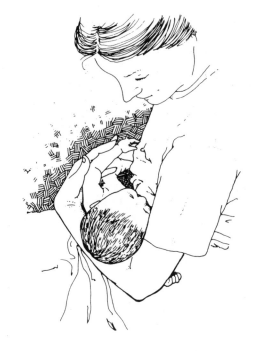

What do you see wrong in this picture with the baby's body position?

The baby's head, neck and back are not in a straight line. The mother should hold the baby across the shoulders, with the neck and back straight, so the baby's head does not tip forward.

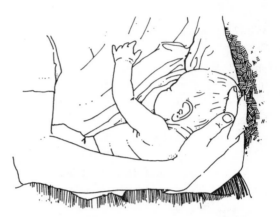

What do you see wrong in this picture about the baby's position?

The baby is lying on his back. In order to feed he will have to turn his head sharply to one side. This will strain his neck. Imagine yourself in his position.

The baby is not tucked in close to his mother's body. It would be difficult for her to bring him close, as his arm is in the way.

What does this woman need to do to correct her baby's position?

She needs to turn her baby towards her, place his lower arm underneath her breast, out of the way, and tuck him in close. Then he will be in a good position to begin to feed.

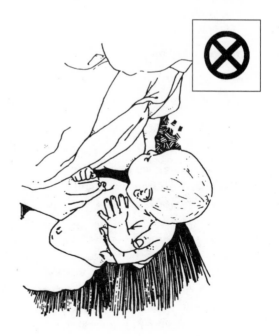

In this drawing you can see clearly how the woman is actually trying to feed her baby her breast, as if her breast were a bottle This will not work and distorts the shape of her breast.

What does this woman need to do differently?

She needs to take him off the breast immediately so that she can try again. She needs to break the suction by placing her finger in the corner of his mouth, and then take him off the breast completely.

Then she needs to think about what it is that she has done and what she needs to do differently. She should go back over the points about good positioning and also read the reminders of what not to do. In this case, she should:

1. place a pillow or something of the right thickness underneath the baby to raise his body up a bit

2. turn his body towards her

3. tuck him in close

4. wait until his mouth gapes widely

5. bring him up onto the breast again

If necessary (if she or the baby is very upset) she would need to calm herself and calm her baby before trying again. Some babies will go on the breast when they are crying, but they will rarely take an adequate mouthful as the tongue is curled back.

Always bring your baby onto your breast, not your breast to your baby.

It is very common today for women to move the breast towards the baby, rather than the baby to the breast (as if they are bottle feeding). Often, even when a woman turns her baby to face her, tucks him in

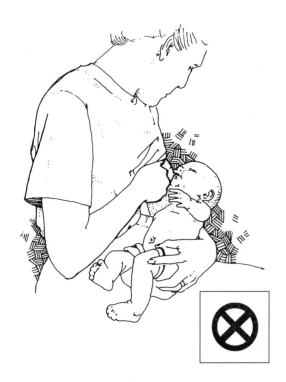

close, makes sure his head is level with her breast and his nose at the level of her nipple, she will then—at the last second—move her body to the baby or move her breast to the baby. If you do this (and it is so commonly done today that we feel it needs to be given special attention) then you will be off to a bad start. If you don't bring your baby onto your breast he will not be able to take a good enough mouthful to protect your nipple and to reach your milk supply. And, once your baby is on the breast and you relax, he will actually be pulling away from your body, stretching your breast, and this will tend to pull the nipple out of his mouth. It is difficult to actually see how much of your breast is in your baby's mouth, you will have to feel it. There are two signs:

1. It should not hurt your nipple, except possibly for a few moments at the beginning.

2. You should feel your baby begin to suckle.

If there is pain in your nipple, and it lasts more than a few seconds, or if you do not feel her starting to feed, then assume that the position of her mouth on your breast is not correct. Gently take her off the breast, take a few relaxing breaths, and begin again.

3. *How your baby takes your breast (see pages 48-53)*

Make sure your baby *takes* your breast; *do not* try to give it to him or push your breast into his mouth.

As your baby goes on your breast, check that he:

- gapes his mouth wide open
- takes a large mouthful of your breast

How to help your baby take your breast:

Position him so that his nose is at the level of your nipple, then when he gapes his mouth it will look like this picture. You will see that when he goes on the breast it is his lower jaw which does the work of taking in a big enough mouthful. His chin should end up pressed against your breast.

Wait until your baby's mouth is beginning to open wide before bringing him onto your breast. If you wait for this to happen, then he will be sure to take a good mouthful—areola and breast tissue as well as nipple. When he takes a good mouthful, your nipple is protected from friction and will not get sore.

Sometimes your baby may open his mouth wide enough by himself. Or you may want to let your nipple brush against his lips or cheek, to show him you are ready. You may need to coax him gently with your voice. See what works for both of you.

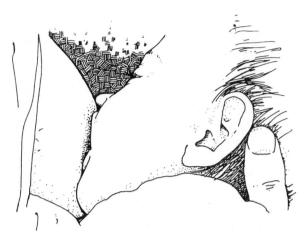

As soon as you see his mouth opening wide, bring it onto your breast with a quick and gentle movement of your hand (or your forearm, if his head is on your forearm).

Here is what your baby should look like when he is feeding. Notice:

1. His chin is against the breast.

2. His mouth is open wide and the lower lip is pressed down and back against his chin.

3. His nose is not touching you breast. You do not need to hold his nose away from your breast.

Note: Some babies may be so close that this is difficult to see.

A Special Note About Pain: There are two sorts of pain you can have when breastfeeding and both can be solved. One is nipple pain. The other is deep breast pain. Nipple pain is due either to poor positioning of the baby's mouth on your breast or a condition called thrush (candida). Deep breast pain can also come from your baby not being well attached to your breast or from thrush. However, if you have pain in the first couple of weeks of feeding it is most likely to be due to damage to your tissue from your baby not being properly on your breast. Good positioning of the baby's mouth on the mother's breast prevents and solves almost all problems women encounter in breastfeeding.

4. How to tell if it's right
(see pages 59-60)

As your baby feeds check that he:

- Sucks strongly and rhythmically, with occasional pauses

- Does not hurt you

- Comes off the breast when he is ready

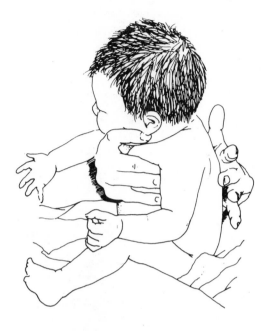

During or after each feed give your baby the chance to burp/wind. You can place the baby on his stomach, over your thigh or on your shoulder. Or you can sit him up, like this, being sure to let his chest rest on your hand and using your top finger to support his chin. Whatever position you use, you do not need to thump your baby on the back. This can actually cause him to spit up all the milk he has taken. You may not need to do anything but sit him upright. Or you may gently rub or pat him on the back.

Your breastfeeding will be going well if your baby:

- Grows steadily

- Has straw-colored (pale yellow or clear), odorless urine

- Has a regular, soft (but not totally liquid) yellow stool (see note that follows)

- Breastfeeds well

A note on your breastfed baby's stools: After the first few days of passing the greenish black meconium stool and then the brown "changing" stool, a baby who is fully breastfed should have a mustard yellow, soft (but not totally liquid) stool. It will look slightly curdled. Babies usually settle into a regular pattern of passing stool. You will soon know your own baby's pattern, and you will see that it gradually changes over time. If there is a sudden change in this pattern (and you have not just changed your baby's diet by introducing other foods), and this change lasts longer than a day or two, watch for any other possible problems. These may be pain in his stomach or a change in color or consistency of the stool.

If all of the signs just listed are present, it is likely that your baby's health and your milk supply are fine.

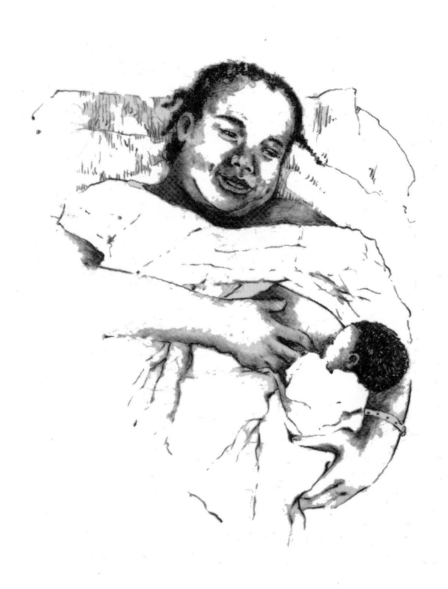

CHAPTER FOUR

Things You Might Need to Know

Low Blood Sugar?

In the past few years, some health professionals and hospitals have started to test breastfed babies routinely to check that they do not have low blood sugar (hypoglycemia). The baby's heel is pricked with a needle to obtain a small sample of blood which is then tested. If the level is lower than the health professional thinks is right, then the baby is offered additional fluids. This may be by offering extra help with breastfeeding, giving expressed colostrum or breast milk, or by giving formula milk or glucose water.

There is no evidence to support such routine testing of all breastfed babies. Low blood sugar can be a problem for some babies, such as babies who are smaller than they are expected to be, who are born prematurely, who become cold, who have an infection, or if the mother is diabetic. These babies and their mothers should receive special attention in the early days of life until feeding is well established. There is no need to test normal, healthy, babies born at term for low blood sugar, as long as they remain healthy; they do not develop signs of low blood sugar simply as a result of underfeeding. It may be that this concern has arisen because of health professionals lack of confidence and experience with breastfeeding over the last few decades.

Breastfeeding well and without restrictions, in the way we have described in this book, will give your baby all that she needs.

Some Practical Hints on Milk Expression

You may need to express your milk for a number of reasons:

- You may have a small or sick baby who cannot breastfeed.

- You may need to be in the hospital and cannot take her with you.

- You may need to be away from your baby longer than an hour or two.

- You may be going back to work where facilities are not available or you do not have the opportunity to breastfeed.

If you have to express a lot of milk regularly, you might want or need to try a hand pump or an electric pump.

There are advantages and disadvantages both to expressing milk by hand to expressing it by pump. Briefly, these include:

1. Hand expression can be done anywhere, anytime, at no cost, with no equipment needed. Some women find they get so skilled with hand expression they do not want to use a pump.

2. Using a good hand or electric pump properly is usually faster than hand expression. A pump that is hard to use, hurts while being used, or makes you feel sore afterward is ineffective and should not be used. If it is possible, try one out before you buy it.

3. Electric pumps are very expensive. Some hospitals rent them out or lend them free of charge to mothers with babies in special care or intensive care units, or if there are major feeding problems. In some countries pump manufacturers have arranged for breastfeeding support groups and lactation consultants to rent out electric pumps. Some pumps provide soft silicone inserts which may or may not help milk expression—try using the pump with and without the insert, to see which works best for you. There are also a number of small electric pumps which are much cheaper.

4. Both hand and electric pumps need to be carefully cleaned after every use. Hand expression requires only basic bodily cleanliness and thorough cleaning of milk containers.

You should decide on your method by seeing which you prefer. We will not discuss hand or electric pumps further here, as other books cover breast pumping adequately (see the resource section). You can sometimes get information about pumps from your local hospital, health workers, or breastfeeding support group. See the resources section (page 203) for help.

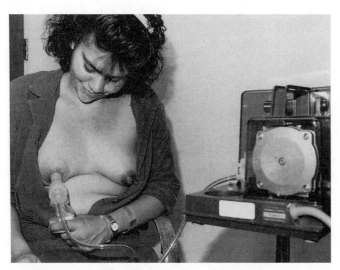

An electric breast pump, like this one, looks imposing but is actually easy to use. Many hospitals have small portable ones that you can borrow and use at home.

This young mother, who has a one-week-old baby who is in the intensive/special care nursery, is able to use the hospitals electric breast pump whenever she wishes. This way her baby can receive her breast milk while he is being tube fed. Take care not to push too hard against your breast while pumping.

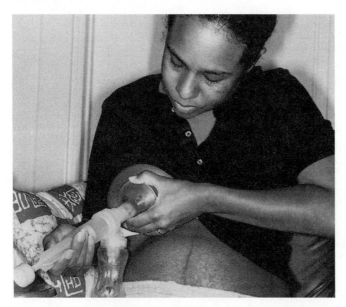

This mother, whose breasts were too full and firm for her small, four-day-old baby to grasp, discovered that using a mechanical breast pump helped. She bought the pump at a pharmacy. By taking a little milk from each breast before a feed, she made her breast softer, and easier for her baby to grasp. She only needed to do this for a few feeds, while she and her baby were getting breastfeeding established. Note how this mother is supporting her breast underneath while pumping.

We will discuss hand expression in detail, because it is free and can be done almost anywhere.

Learning to Hand Express

Many women find hand expression messy and frustrating at first. Like everything else to do with breastfeeding, practice makes it easy.

It is helpful to know that you can do this easily, without equipment, in case of emergency. *Practice it a few times before you need it.* Trying to express in a hurry before you leave your baby for the first time is not the best way to learn. Visualize this as a time to feed your baby, even if she cannot be with you. Set time aside as if your were settling down to feed.

Expressing in a warm bath or shower the first few times you try might help. The warm water is relaxing, and you don't have to think about what to do with the milk. Concentrate on the expression at first, rather than catching the milk. Use some tissues or a clean cloth to catch the milk if you are not in the bath or shower. Express before a feed, rather than after; there is more milk and expression is easier.

You might find, like many women, that if you gently massage your breast first, lightly stroking down with your hand toward the nipple for a few minutes, the milk will flow more easily.

The pictures here show you the details of expression. Note that the mother is learning while her baby is on her lap. This often makes expression easier, as your letdown reflex is more likely to work well (see page 68). If you cannot hold your baby or if she is not there to look at, try holding something else that reminds you of her or relaxes you: a blanket, a stuffed animal, your older child, whatever helps.

Many women find it helps to look at a photograph of the baby. If your baby is in a special care or intensive care unit, the staff will be happy for you to arrange to have a picture taken of your baby. Some will do it for you. (You might also tape a photograph of yourself and your family to your baby's bed in the hospital to remind the staff that your baby is part of a family.)

You can use either hand on either breast. Most women use the same hand for both breasts; their choice of hand may depend on whether they are right-handed or lefthanded.

There are many different ways of getting milk out of the breast. Each mother adapts the basics to suit her body. We give you just one description of how to get your milk flowing; you'll discover other ways for yourself as you become more confident.

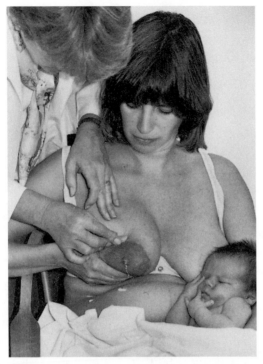

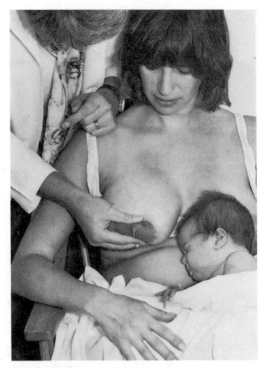

When you are learning to express, have your baby with you, if possible, as this will help your milk release.

If it is not possible for your baby to be with you, then try cuddling something else—an older child, a special object—or look at a picture of your baby.

It helps to have a skilled person to teach you. If you do not have someone, then practice using the description here. Remember the milk supply is well back behind your nipple.

Place your thumb flat against the upper edge of your areola and cup the rest of your hand under your breast with the lower fingers against your ribs.

Gently squeeze your thumb and forefinger together, while at the same time pressing your whole hand back and in toward your breast, to reach the milk.

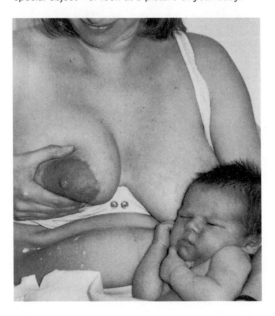

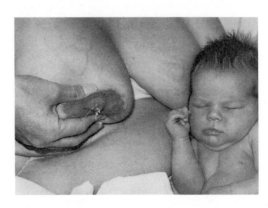

1. Place your thumb flat on the upper edge of your areola, and cup the rest of your hand under your breast with your three lower fingers against your ribs.

   To do this well you need to have a good handful of breast between your thumb and the rest of your hand. Feel the weight of your breast in your cupped hand. If you have a small areola, then move your fingers farther apart than the edge of your areola. If your areola is large, then move your fingers in a bit toward your nipple.

2. Imagine that milk is coming from deep within the breast through tiny holes. Rather than pinching the tubes closed, you want to push the milk along and out. To do this, gently squeeze your thumb and forefinger together. At the same time gently press your whole hand back and in, toward your chest.

   You need to do both these steps *together*, so that you milk the deep breast tissue as well as squeezing milk out of the ducts that lie right under the nipple and areola.

   The resulting movement should feel like you are *pressing back in toward yourself*, and then releasing again, rather than squeezing.

   Just as your baby makes his milking action with his lower jaw, most of the work is not in your thumb, but in the part of the hand that is supporting your breast.

   Some people like to think of keeping the thumb stationary while doing all the work with the lower fingers. Think of bringing the lower fingers up toward the thumb and folding your breast up, thus releasing the stream of milk.

   Whichever way you do it, be careful not to slide your thumb or forefinger over your skin toward your nipple. This can cause a burning sensation. Don't be rough with your breasts: they bruise easily. Expressing should not hurt.

   Once you have the movement right, your milk may take up to a minute or two to flow. Keeping repeating the movement until you feel confident.

When you start to collect milk, simply hold a wide-mouthed container under the flow of milk. Some women have an active letdown reflex and find that the milk flow is rapid and shoots a few inches away from the nipple.

Storage of Breast Milk

Today in the United States, women are rarely advised to sterilize equipment. It may be that you live where you have clean water and clean surroundings, then you do not need to sterilize. But it is our belief that it is best to sterilize all milk containers, storage jars, and feeding utensils, by boiling them for ten minutes. A sterilizing solution or steam sterilizer may also be used; the manufacturer's instructions should be followed. If you do not sterilize, then wash everything very carefully with hot, soapy water and and rinse off the soap thoroughly. A final scalding with just-boiled water may also help.

Once you have expressed your milk, look after it carefully. If it stays at room temperature, you should use it almost immediately. It will keep in a refrigerator for two or three days. In a separate freezer it can keep for a month. If you have a small freezing space within your refrigerator, do not keep it there longer than two weeks. Do not store breast milk in the rack in the refrigerator or freezer door; keep it at the back, where it is coldest.

Never refreeze milk after it has thawed, and remember not to use a microwave oven to thaw or warm frozen milk. A microwave does not heat evenly. It can over-heat the milk in the center of the container and scald the baby! It also destroys vitamin C, and some studies suggest it may alter proteins.

Inverted Nipples and Nipples that Do Not Stand Out (Flat)

It is not uncommon for a woman to have one or both nipples that dip inward, like a crater, rather than stand out. These are called inverted nipples. It is also normal for a woman to have one or both nipples that do not stand out when she is cold, sexually aroused, or starting to breastfeed. These are called flat (or nonprotractile) nipples.

It is possible to breastfeed with either of these kinds of nipples, although it will be more difficult at the beginning, and you will need patience, understanding of what to do, and probably some help.

Remember that babies do not nipple feed: they breastfeed! So right from the very first feed, encourage your baby to take a large moutful of breast, as we describe on page 51. As your baby feeds from your breast, he will draw the nipple out by his sucking action.

You may find it helpful to stimulate your nipples with your fingers just before feeding, to help them stand out. Some women like to express some milk before a feed, so that the baby gets milk as soon as he starts to suck.

Some people advise that women with inverted or flat nipples prepare their breasts in pregnancy. Two treatments are described: glass or plastic breast shells that fit over the nipple and part of the breast and are worn inside the bra, and exercises to stretch the base of the nipple, using the thumbs or forefingers (Hoffman's exercises). Neither of these treatments work. If either of them are carried out too vigorously, there is a possibility of damage to the nipples.

If you have problems with your baby taking your breast, and you cannot solve them, don't panic. The best thing to do is to express your milk from the side (or sides) that is causing the problem, and feed your milk to your baby by spoon, cup, or bottle (see pages 101-102).

Many women find that as their babies get bigger, it becomes easier for them to feed from inverted or nonprotractile nipples. So you might find that you express for two or three weeks, and then your baby is able to breastfeed. In this instance you may have to persist for a few days to teach him to take your breast, because he will not be used to opening his mouth wide to feed.

If you have difficulty with one breast only, it is perfectly possible to breastfeed successfully from only one side, and either express milk or not feed at all from the other side. Over time, your milk supply will adjust to your baby's needs, so that one breast will provide all the milk he needs. See the case study on pages 179-180 for an example of how easy this can be.

A Word About Your Diet

While you are breastfeeding, what you eat is important. In pregnancy your baby was growing inside you, and you were aware that you needed to eat well to help him grow and develop healthily. During breastfeeding, your baby is growing fast and depends entirely on the milk you are making.

Your body is surprisingly efficient at making milk. In fact, it seems to conserve energy, becoming far more efficient than usual during the time you were breastfeeding. So you don't really need to eat for two.

But you need to force yourself to eat well to ensure that you have enough protein, vitamins, calories (carbohydrates and fats), and minerals for both your needs and your baby's growth. Regular meals are necessary; either two large meals each day or frequent snacks throughout the day, containing plenty of fresh fruits and vegetables. You can breastfeed successfully if you are a vegetarian, but do ask your health worker for advice.

Avoid dieting during this time. You will be surprised how easily you lose the extra weight from pregnancy while you breastfeed; this is one of the advantages of breastfeeding. And it looks as if the hormones you release while breastfeeding actually help you to lose weight from the buttocks and thighs, usually the most difficult places to reduce.

Contary to popular opinion, you do not need to drink extra fluids while you are breastfeeding. Many women find, however, that they are especially thirsty, and it is always wise to respond to your body's needs. Simply drink a glass of water, juice, or other beverage whenever you are thirsty. It is a good idea to have a glass of something to drink by your side before you settle down to breastfeed.

Your baby will essentially be taking in small amounts of whatever substances you take in. Think carefully about your intake of nicotine, sugar, and artificial sweeteners. Think especially carefully about your alcohol and caffeine (found in chocolate and many teas and soft drinks as well as coffee) intake. They pass quickly into the breast milk and affect the baby in the same way they affect you. Having these substances occasionally is fine, but regular or heavy intake will affect your baby.

Some women become so busy and preoccupied that they forget to eat or drink regularly. Neglecting your needs is not difficult to do when you are caring for the needs of a young baby, and perhaps other children as well. If this happens to you, remember that it can harm your health. You will probably continue to make enough milk, but you will become very tired. Ask others to remind you to eat, and keep food that is easy to prepare in the house. Do remember to drink whenever you are thirsty.

Taking Drugs or Medications While Breastfeeding

During the time you are breastfeeding, you must continue to be as careful about taking medications or drugs as you were during pregnancy. Anything you take will cross into your breast milk. Even drugs you consider harmless, such as aspirin, may have an effect on the baby. It is surprising how often we take tablets when we don't need them.

Follow this principle: *If you do not have to take a drug or medication, don't.* This warning includes drugs like marijuana or cocaine. There are no safe levels of these drugs for babies.

Alcohol, caffeine, and tobacco are drugs too, all of which directly affect the breastfeeding baby. See the section on diet (pages 92-93). Breastfeeding women who smoke are more likely to have babies who cry and develop "colic." And alcohol passes quickly into the breast milk. It has the same effect on babies as it has on us, and is harmful in regular or large doses. An occasional drink is fine, but not more.

If you have to take medication, make sure your doctor knows that you are breastfeeding, and ask her or him to explain the possible effects on the baby. Many drugs are compatible with breastfeeding. For example, if you are diabetic and take insulin every day, you can certainly continue to breastfeed. But make sure your doctor knows you are breastfeeding and helps you adjust your insulin dose accordingly.

We cannot list in this book the possible side effects of each drug. In fact, much research is still needed examining the effects of drugs or medications on breastfed babies. An easy-to-read book lists commonly used drugs and their possible effects when taken during pregnancy and lactation. You will find it listed in "Books You Might Find Helpful" on page 220. A good bookshop should be able to order it for you.

If You Also Have Other Children to Care For

Spending time with your new baby and working out how to get feeding right can be challenging, especially if you have a feeding problem which needs your time and attention. If you have other children, especially a toddler, this can be very difficult. You have to deal with the older child or children's emotional reactions to the new baby: they may be jealous, or pleased or proud (or all of these at different times). They may become very interested and want to play with the baby, so that they disturb him whenever he is settled. Or they may ignore him altogether.

If you have others to help you, a partner or a neighbor or friends, you may be able to find a quiet place for your baby when he needs to be fed, and also find time to pay special attention to your toddler at another time during the day. Do ask for help at this time; people are often delighted to be asked to help a new mother.

If you are on your own much of the time, and find you need to concentrate on feeding in the early days before it becomes easy, you will need to be creative and work out ways of keeping your toddler entertained. Toddlers seem to be expert at interrupting feeds by wanting something to eat, poking the baby, asking for the potty or doing things that are dangerous or forbidden in order to get your attention.

It is worth thinking ahead. Find ways of making feeding times special for your toddler too. Allow her to do things she especially likes at these times. Try some of the following when you start to breastfeed:

- make sure the room is as childproof as possible, and move all dangerous or fragile objects out of reach.

- Give her a drink and treat like a biscuit or cookies, chopped fruit or raisins

- Put on a story or music tape, or a video

- Take out a box of toys you have put away for special occasions

- Keep the potty close at hand where you can reach it

- Give her a doll and encourage her to breastfeed it just like you

- Ask an older child to play with the younger one

If you can, spend time with your toddler soon *after* the baby is settled, to cuddle and reassure her that she can still have her special times with you too. Also spend time with her when the baby is asleep. Your toddler is likely to have a nap in the daytime too, and you may be able to use this time to be with your baby or to take a well deserved nap yourself. Even just lying down and having your feet up helps.

Remember that this stage *will* pass, that feeding will become easier, and that she *will* become accustomed to the baby and to feeding times.

You may find yourself feeling that you cannot cope, or becoming very angry with your toddler, if feeding is difficult and her behavior very challenging. You may find yourself doing things you would normally not do; letting her watch more television than you would normally like, giving her more treats than usual. Don't worry; once you have all settled down, you can change these things back to normal. It is important that you *all* have the time to adjust to a situation that is challenging for all of you.

If You Are Ill

If you become ill, *do your best to keep your milk supply stimulated*. During the time you are sick, *make rest and breastfeeding your priorities*. You can arrange for help around the house and go to bed if necessary, taking your baby with you. Then you can both simply rest and breastfeed.

If you need to be admitted to the hospital, try to arrange to have your baby stay with you. Sometimes you can share a room so you can be together. If your baby cannot come with you and you are well enough, express your milk regularly and send it home. If you are not well enough to do this yourself, ask your health workers or family members to help you. Remember that the painful engorgement and mastitis that could occur if you suddenly stop breastfeeding will not help your recovery.

If you do have to stop breastfeeding for a while or if your milk simply decreases, *it is always possible to restart or increase your supply.* See the section on relactation (page 103). If you have to take medications, read the section on drugs and breastfeeding (page 93).

If Your Baby Has Special Needs

If a baby is born with a physical problem, parents become very distressed, especially the first few days after birth. At this time, it is hard to think clearly and to plan for the baby's feeding. Many babies with special needs can breastfeed, and sometimes breastfeeding can even help.

When a baby is born with special needs it is common for health workers to want to observe the baby carefully. In many cases this means separating the infant from his mother. If a health worker suggests that your baby needs to be in the special care or intensive care unit, question whether his separation from you is necessary. Make your desires to be with your baby known. If you must be separated, start to express your milk soon after birth (see pages 86-90). You may find the section of special care or intensive care helpful (see page 98-100).

If your baby has special needs, it will be valuable to contact other parents who have dealt with the same challenge. Many parent support groups exist, both at the local and national level. Addresses for some groups are listed in "Where to Find Help" (see page 203). Your local health workers or breastfeeding support group will be able to put you in touch with the group nearest you.

These are the principles which apply to breastfeeding any baby with special needs:

- *Be determined that your baby will have breast milk*, whether it is from your breast or by tube, bottle, spoon, or cup. The health-giving properties of breast milk, including the increased resistance to infection that it provides, are especially important for babies.

- *Work with your baby to help him take your breast.* Find support and skilled assistance to help you.

- Even if you cannot feed from your breast, *have lots of skin-to-skin contact with your baby.*

Three of the most common conditions with which babies are born are Down's syndrome (sometimes called mongolism), cleft lip and/or palate, and heart defects. We will discuss these here.

Babies born with Down's syndrome have decreased muscle tone, so they find it harder to support their own heads. Their bodies also have to be supported more than those of other babies. But once they have learned to feed from the breast, they can breastfeed well; and both mother and baby will benefit from the health advantages of breastfeeding and from the close contact. It helps greatly to be in touch with other parents who have faced the same situation. Contact your breastfeeding support group or a support group for parents with Down's syndrome babies; addresses are provided in "Where to Find Help."

Babies who have cleft lip can usually breastfeed. It is unlikely that babies with a cleft palate will be able to breastfeed effectively. Even if feeding from your breast is not possible, you can feed your baby expressed breast milk, making it possible for him to grow and thrive on your milk.

Babies with a cleft palate will find it hard to suck and swallow efficiently. You could try to feed with your baby in a semi-upright position and stop frequently to give him time to cope with the milk flow. Ask for advice from your health worker, breastfeeding support group, or cleft palate association (see "Where to Find Help"). If you find it difficult to feed from your breast, or if you cannot provide all your baby's needs this way, you can express your milk and feed your baby using a bottle and teat designed for babies with clefts. Again, ask your health worker or support group for more information.

Even if you cannot feed from your breast, you can still cuddle your baby against your breast. In this way, your baby will have the advantages of drinking your breast milk from a bottle and of being close to you. Some babies with clefts will have surgery when they are slightly older to correct it. Breast milk is the best way to ensure that your baby is healthy for the surgery, and cuddling is the way to keep him happy.

Babies with heart defects can also be breastfed. Recent information suggests that breastfeeding does not stress babies as much as bottle feeding. It is harder work to suck and swallow from a bottle than from the breast. So breastfeeding may be especially advantageous for babies with heart problems who need to conserve their energy as much as possible.

Jenny's story, in "Women's Breastfeeding Stories" (page 174), shows how one mother, with support from her family and health workers, successfully managed a baby with a particularly severe heart problem.

Remember, breastfeeding a baby with special needs is especially valuable. He needs the health-giving properties of breast milk, and the close contact and cuddles will comfort you both.

If Your Baby Is in the Special Care or Intensive Care Unit

If your baby is in the special care or intensive care nursery for any reason, you will want to have as much contact as you can with him. It is especially important for both of you that you start and then maintain a good milk supply.

Breast milk from their own mothers is almost always the best food, by far, for small or sick babies. In spite of the many advantages of breastfeeding for these babies, it can be difficult to do. The routines in some special care or intensive care units are not supportive of breastfeeding. The units themselves can be noisy, crowded, and hot, and it can be hard to find a chair or get to your baby's bedside so that you can calmly touch and stroke (or just be with) your baby.

Find support from helpers who believe that your presence and breastfeeding are best for your baby. Then persist patiently, because the more your baby grows, the easier breastfeeding will become.

In summary,

- Have as much contact as possible with your baby. Cuddle him skin to skin if you can. Hold his hand or foot, or stroke him in the incubator. (If you can do nothing else, simply be with him and let him hear the sound of your voice reassuring him that all is well.)

- Start to express your milk soon after birth, and express your milk again every two or three hours after that (see pages 86-90), just as if he were with you and breastfeeding. Include a nighttime expression of milk if you possibly can.

- If you cannot be with your baby while you express milk, look at a photograph of him, or cuddle something else—a soft toy, a blanket, your older child.

- Express each time for only as long as is comfortable (or until the milk stops flowing). Remember to gently massage your breast before you begin, and don't express for so long that you get sore.

- Ask the hospital staff if they lend electric breast pumps for use at home; it can save time if you are having to express often throughout the day.

- Tape a photograph of you and your family to your baby's crib in the hospital, so that the staff know who you all are and remember to think of your baby as part of a family.

- Ask the staff about arrangements for storage and collection of your breast milk.

- Don't worry if you get only a small amount of milk when you first begin to express it. Keep expressing frequently to build up your supply. A baby is more efficient at getting milk than you are at expressing milk.

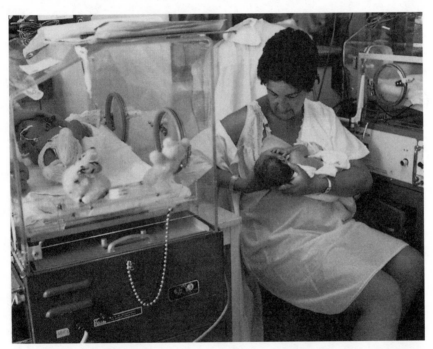

It is difficult to begin breastfeeding with your baby in an intensive care unit (special care baby unit). But breastfeeding, or providing breast milk for your baby, is the best thing you can do for your baby at this time. Be patient. Be persistent. Ask for whatever help you need, and keep asking if you don't get an answer that works. Take all the time you and your baby need to learn to get it right.

- When you first try to breastfeed, take your time, be patient with yourself and your baby, and have an understanding helper nearby. Don't be disappointed if the baby does not feed immediately. He may relax so completely in your arms that he just falls asleep.

A very small baby can be sleepy and need a bit of stimulation to get interested in feeding. It will become easier for both of you as your confidence develops and your baby gets bigger.

- Take care with positioning.

- Do not rush putting your baby onto the breast.

- Let your baby feed for as long as he wants.

- If your baby stops for a while, see if he needs to burp or wind, and then continue.

Above all, be patient! And ask for help *whenever* you need it. You *can* breastfeed well, even with a small or sick baby.

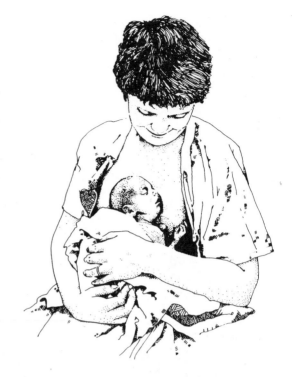

All babies love skin to skin contact, but it is especially valuable for sick or small babies.

When You Cannot Feed Your Baby from Your Breast

If you cannot feed from your breast, either for a few feeds or a few weeks, you can feed your milk to your baby in a number of ways.

If your baby is small or sick, he may need to be tube fed. The hospital staff will advise you on caring for him. The best food for him is your breast milk, even if you cannot feed it to him yourself.

Bottles are the most common way of giving feeds to babies, but they are not the only way. If a baby is small or has feeding problems, it may confuse him to give him a bottle teat. A baby does not have to open his mouth as widely to take in a bottle teat as he does to take in a breast.

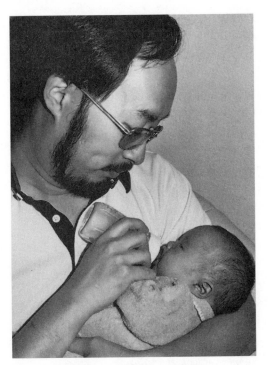

No matter how you are feeding your baby, be sure to cuddle him in close to your body. Feeding, for a baby, is as much about human contact and touch as it is about nourishment.

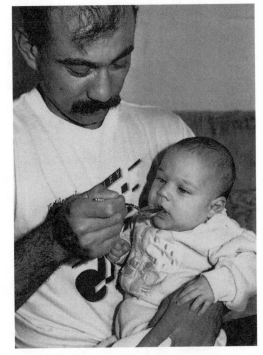

You can feed even a very young baby by spoon. When she starts making sucking movements, tilt the spoon a little and the milk will go in. She doesn't need much of a mouthful.

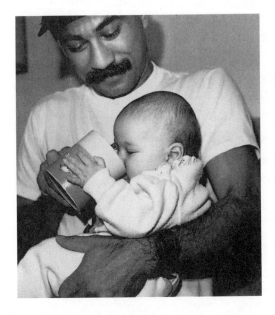

This father is feeding his three-month-old daughter from a cup.

If you want to use a cup, bring it to your baby's lips, tilt it so that just a tiny amount of fluid goes into her mouth. Feed her very slowly, giving her a chance to swallow each mouthful.

You (or your partner or helper) can feed your baby by using a cup or small glass. Simply put a small amount of milk in the cup or glass and gently tilt it to your baby's lips (see picture on page 101). Watch carefully and feed slowly. It does work!

Similarly, you can feed by spoon. Use a teaspoon and put a small amount of milk on it. Place the spoon gently against the baby's lips. When he starts to make sucking movements, tilt the spoon a little and the milk will go in. You can also try using a small dropper and gently drop milk into your baby's mouth. Be careful to do this very slowly, and watch for him to swallow before you put more in.

Whichever way you choose to feed, remember that your baby needs lots of contact with you while you do it. For both adult and baby, the experience is quite different: cuddles and food are both important.

Breastfeeding an Adopted Baby

It is possible to breastfeed an adopted baby. Though it is unlikely you will be able to stimulate your milk supply to fully breastfeed, *you can put your baby to your breast, enjoy her feeding, and your breasts will be stimulated to make some milk, even if you have never been pregnant or breastfed before.*

It will be beneficial to talk with your health worker or breastfeeding support group. Since breastfeeding an adopted baby is not always easy, it is useful to have support from someone who has seen it done or done it herself. If you cannot find help, the general principles are:

- Make sure your baby has enough food. You can feed her by bottle, cup, spoon, or breastfeeding supplementer (see below) while you work on starting your milk supply.

- Never put her to your breast if she is very hungry, because she will become frustrated and cry. You both should associate the breast with pleasure. If she is hungry, feed her a little to calm her before putting her to your breast.

- Put your baby to your breast and let her suckle as often as you can. Pay careful attention to positioning to avoid soreness and to teach her to breastfeed properly (see pages 45-53). She probably will be used to bottle feeding, and the suckling action at the breast is different.

- Let her suckle on each breast for as long and as often as she wants. She will enjoy the cuddling and sucking, and you will have the pleasure of feeling her close to you. Stop and check your positioning if it is painful for you.

- Some women find that using a breastfeeding supplementer is helpful. This is a container for milk (either artificial milk or expressed breast milk), attached to a fine plastic tube which you can tape close to your nipple. As the baby feeds at your breast, she also feeds, through the tube, from the container. For suppliers, see the addresses on page 203, or contact your local breastfeeding support group.

- It will take some weeks for your milk supply to respond. But during this time, you and your baby will have the pleasure of closeness that is not possible if you simply feed her from the bottle. Remember that breastfeeding is much more than a way to feed your baby; it is a way to give love and comfort too.

Relactating: Starting the Breastfeed After Having Stopped

You may have stopped breastfeeding and then decided you want to start again. Perhaps you were advised to stop and now find that you should have been able to breastfeed after all. Maybe you and your baby were separated for some reason and are now together; or, after weaning, your baby has become sick and you want to feed her breast milk again. You may have found that you simply miss breastfeeding.

You will be able to restart your milk supply. Most women find that even months after they stop breastfeeding they can still express some milk. It is possible to increase that supply by feeding regularly. To begin breastfeeding again, you simply put your baby to your breast as often and for as long as you can. Obviously, you will need to make sure she has enough to eat while your milk supply responds. And be careful with positioning; don't continue to feed if it hurts you. The guidelines for relactating are similar to those for breastfeeding an adopted baby, but your supply will respond much more quickly. Some women find that using a breastfeeding supplementer is helpful (see above).

What About Weaning?

Note: Weaning means different things in different countries. It may mean the introduction of solid foods, or it may mean the cessation of breastfeeding. In this section we are referring to the introduction of solid foods. At the end we will discuss stopping breastfeeding

It is best if you can feed your baby entirely on breast milk for the first six months. This gives the baby the best nutrition as well as protection from infection and from developing sensitivity to other foods. Many women continue to breast-feed exclusively for longer than 6 months and some babies continue to thrive on breast milk alone until they are 9 months old. But by this stage, many babies need to have a more varied diet. Be guided by your own feelings and your baby's health and appetite.

You can start to give your baby extra fluids or food while continuing to breast-feed. In fact some women breastfeed for over two years. They feed their babies solids and other fluids, but also breastfeed once or more a day for as long as both they as their babies want to continue.

Whether you start to give your baby other fluids or food at two or at six months, the general principle is to do it gradually. This will help your baby adjust to new foods. Equally important, it prevents you from becoming engorged. It is possible to develop mastitis if you get very full, which may happen for a few days as you cut down on breastfeeding, so watch carefully for signs of redness and pain in your breasts (see page 117).

Your baby is used to receiving all of her food from you. Some breastfed babies do not like to take bottles or food from a spoon. *Be patient and creative.* If she refuses a bottle, try something else. If you introduce food gradually and continue to breastfeed, you will feel no pressure to force her to eat more than she desires or needs.

If she does not like the new food or if she becomes sick for any reason and refuses to eat, one of the advantages of breastfeeding is that you can return to full breastfeeding. Simply stop giving her the extra food or fluids and let her feed from your breast as often as she likes. Your milk supply will respond in a day or two, and you can continue to breastfeed until she has recovered from her illness. Then you can start introducing new foods again, but remember to do it gradually.

If you need to cut down or stop breastfeeding before six months, to go back to work or for any other reason, the next best thing to breast milk is formula milk. This is modified milk for babies which can be bought in most food and drug-stores. Some countries supply free or subsidized formula milk for women with low incomes. Ask your health worker for further information.

Do not be tempted to give your baby ordinary cows' milk, especially not low fat or skimmed milk. Because babies grow quickly, they must have the right bal-ance of fat, protein and minerals. Ordinary cow's milk (or goat's milk) does not meet a human infants' needs, and your baby may get sick if you give this to her.

Keep all bottles, spoon and cups clean: even when babies are older they can still pick up infections if cleanliness is neglected.

As soon as you introduce food or fluids other than breast milk, your baby's bowel habits will change. Her stool, which has been sweet smelling and yellow while breastfeeding, will become firmer, darker, and more smelly. Check that she does not develop diarrhea or constipation after introducing new foods.

When introducing any new food to your baby, start with small amounts (just a teaspoon or two at a meal). Don't be tempted to give her more, even if she seems to be enjoying it. Some babies may be sensitive or allergic to new food, and it is important to watch for signs of distress throughout the 24 hours after introducing a food. Watch for more frequent crying, more wind or gas, or a skin rash anywhere. If all is well, give her more at each feeding.

Introduce only one new food at a time, especially if your family has a history of allergic reactions to certain foods. If you give her two or three new foods at once and she becomes

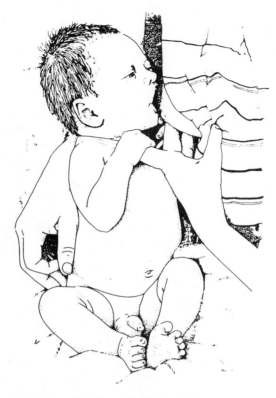

This is a drawing of an older baby, who has learned to turn towards the breast. A new baby would need his or her body tucked closely into the mother's.

distressed, you will not know which food caused the problem. At first avoid foods that you or the baby's father are allergic to. It is possible that your baby will be sensitive to the same foods, so introduce these foods slowly and carefully.

The best guide for weaning your baby is her response to new foods. You and your baby both need to try things out and see how each responds. Do not force her to eat foods she does not like, and gradually work toward feeding her as wide a variety of foods as you can.

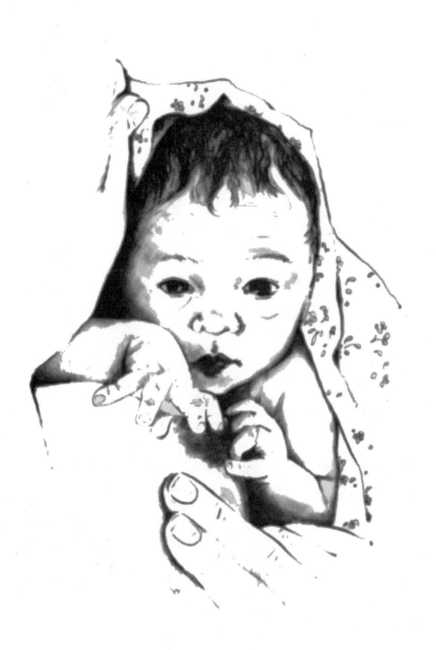

CHAPTER FIVE

Problems: Their Causes and Solutions

*R*ead *this introduction only when you feel calm and your baby is not cry-ing. If you need to know about a problem you have right now, turn to the list on page 114 for immediate help.*

Most problems with breastfeeding can either be prevented or easily treated. If a problem arises, you should try to find the cause. If you treat only the symptoms, then the problem may happen again or even get worse. Some problems may occur in the early days of breastfeeding, others after you have been breastfeeding for some time. Some breastfeeding problems occur in Western countries so often that people think they are inevitable. Babies who cry for long periods and sore nipples are two examples of this. Other problems are uncommon, and people may tell you that they cannot be solved.

We believe all breastfeeding problems have causes. With understanding and skill, almost all problems can be solved. If you find breastfeeding is difficult or stressful for you or your baby, it is likely that you do have a problem. It is also likely that you can fix it. Remember that even when you are working on solving a problem, you are still continuing to breastfeed, and you are still giving your baby the best possible start in life. Some women continue to breastfeed for months even though they have problem, but it's obviously more pleasant for you and your baby if you can solve them.

Don't give up breastfeeding without a fight. The majority of both common and uncommon problems can be solved. But it will take knowledge, understanding, and patience.

One problem can quickly lead to another, just as in birth one intervention, such as induction of labor, can lead to another. For example, a problem with position-ing may result in engorgement or a crying baby or sore nipples—or all three at once! It is important to try to prevent problems from multiplying in this way, and to treat any problem as fast as possible.

It is always better to have someone to help you when you are trying to solve problems. If the steps recommended here do not help you solve your problem on your own, then seek help from the best available source. This may be the local breast-feeding support group, a health worker, or a lactation consultant. If you cannot find good help nearby, check the sources of information listed in the resource section.

This section will tell you how to recognize both common and unusual problems and how to solve them.

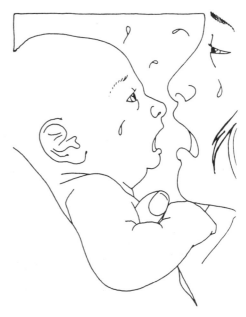

If you get frustrated and your baby gets upset, stop trying. Calm yourself. Calm your baby. Breathe slowly. Then try again.

Home Remedies

Every culture has home remedies for illnesses of all kinds. Many are still widely used, having been passed from generation to generation by word of mouth. May people find various home remedies helpful. The use of home reme-dies is a valuable part of caring for yourself and your baby, both for prevention and treatment of problems.

A home remedy is different from many of the standard products that can be bought in a pharmacy, but some over-the-counter drugs are actually botanical preparations derived from traditional home remedies. An example is senna, the plant that has been used for centuries to treat constipation and is now a major ingredient in many popular laxatives.

Home remedies can include herbal preparations, homeopathic remedies, vita-min and mineral supplements, as well as hands-on care like massage and heat therapy. Some have gained wide acceptance. For example, in many European and Latin American countries, the common found herbs mint and chamomile are reg-ularly used for digestive ailments and whenever a sedative is needed, including treating colic in babies.

Colostrum and breast milk are used as home remedies for the treatment of several common breastfeeding problems. Some women express colostrum and spread it on sore nipples during the first days of breastfeeding (of course, we are suggesting you need not have sore nipples in the first place). Some professionals recommend the use of colostrum or breast milk as a treatment for sticky eyes in newborn babies. One home remedy that is well accepted by the general public and health workers alike for treatment of mastitis is bed rest and an ample intake of fluids.

Home remedies differ markedly from culture to culture. For example, in Western thought many people swear by alternating repeating applications of heat and cold for swelling and injuries of all kinds, including breast engorgement. Warm compresses are applied for half an hour, then ice packs. Chinese wisdom never recommends the use of cold, for either external application or in the form of food or drink, because of their belief that cold has a depressing effect on the body's energy system. In Japan fresh ginger root, grated and dropped into a large pot of boiling water, is used in hot compresses for swelling and infections of all kinds, including breast engorgement, plugged ducts, and breast infection. A treatment now prescribed in Australia by the mainstream medical community that derived from folk wisdom is the use of raw cabbage leaves held against the breast to relieve engorgement.

Scientific evidence from human or animal studies suggests that a number of home remedies may have real medical efficacy and are perfectly safe. However, there is rarely *enough* evidence to make a solid recommendation for their use. Often, little or no good research has been conducted to investigate these remedies; scientists may not know about the existence of such practices or, even when they are aware of them, may not perceive them to be of high enough priority to study.

Home remedies may take longer than prescription drugs to correct a medical problem. They often require more time and effort on your part. Some people may find them helpful, while others won't. One problem with home remedies is the question of what is the right dosage for you or you baby.

At best, a home remedy saves you money and a visit to a health worker and prevents the need for prescription drugs. For example, bed rest, fluids, and continued breastfeeding as an early treatment for mastitis is an alternative to treating mastitis with antibiotics. Antibiotics, though fast and effective, change the body's natural balance and may result in a yeast infection that will require yet another prescription drug.

Some home remedies, like vitamin C and echinacea (a common homeopathic remedy that is also the basis of a popular herbal tincture) are believed to boost the immune system and thereby aid the body's own healing response. Others that had been though to be useful for many ailments have been proven to have negative side effects, especially if taken in large doses, such as comfrey when taken internally.

At worst, a home remedy may not work at all, may do some harm, or may delay you from getting necessary medical treatment. So, if you do try any home remedy, watch carefully for signs of improvement in yourself or your baby. Be prepared to contact a local health worker if you see no signs of improvement or if new symptoms appear. We have only recommended the use of a few remedies that we feel have been tested and found to be both safe and effective.

If you are interested in the use of home remedies, ask around and be sure to check into possible side effects and proper dosages. Be careful, just as you would with the use of prescription drugs. You must be the judge of what sort of treatment you choose for yourself and for your baby. It is important to know that problems that arise in breastfeeding can quickly become more serious if they are not treated. This may occur when the woman or her health worker doesn't recognize the condition as a problem or because the proper treatment is not clear. In addition women often find it hard to take time to look after themselves, especially when they have a young baby and possibly other children or a job to handle as well.

One final warning: babies who are sick or are losing weight or showing other signs such as severe vomiting or diarrhea should receive attention from a health worker.

A World About Blame

 Problems with breastfeeding can be frustrating and painful. They are also deeply emotional.

Breastfeeding problems like sore nipples or a constantly crying baby or a baby who doesn't gain weight can challenge your feelings about yourself, your feelings about your baby, and your confidence in yourself. These problems can put stress on your relationship with your partner, and they can get in the way of developing a relationship with your baby.

We have observed that a common reaction to these deep feelings is to look for something or someone to blame. This blaming may be conscious or unconscious. It is always unhelpful.

It helps to know that this might happen, and to watch for signs of blame from other people. You might even feel a need to blame yourself sometimes.

Be careful. *Do not let people blame you, your baby, or nature for any*
problems. Problems can almost always be solved, and they always have a cause
that can be explained.

Do Not Blame Yourself

You might be told that the problem is your fault because:

• Your are too anxious, inhibited, or uptight

• You did not prepare your nipples

• You don't really want to breastfeed anyway

• Your breasts or nipples are the wrong size or shape

• You don't know enough about breastfeeding

• You are continuing in spite of your baby's problems because you are doing it
for your own sake

None of these is likely to be the case.

Do Not Blame Your Baby

It is sometimes tempting to think that the problem is deliberately caused by
your newborn baby. You may be told that your baby:

• Is *angry*, when in fact she is hungry and frustrated

• Is *lazy*, when in fact she is too tired, jaundiced, sleeping from drugs, or hungry
to feed well

• Is *demanding*, when in fact she is crying from hunger and the need for comfort

• Has an *aggressive suck*, when in fact your nipples are damaged from positioning problems and your baby is hungry

This is all counterproductive and untrue.

Do Not Blame Nature

Some people may blame your body for not producing the right quality or
quantity of milk. Their unspoken message is that there is a basic design flaw in
women's bodies, in spite of all the evidence that the human race survived surprisingly well before bottles were invented. Women today still succeed in breastfeeding wherever bottles and artificial milk are not available.

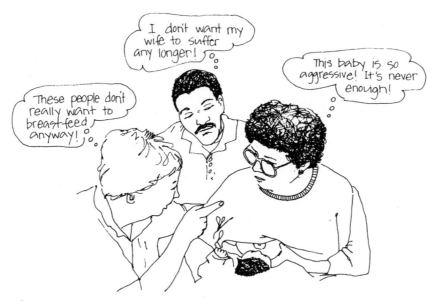

Everyone has an opinion and it's so easy to blame.

Be careful of people who tell you that:

- Your milk is too thin
- You don't have enough milk (although only a very few women really do not have enough, many women are told that this is the case)
- You have too much milk
- Your milk is too rich
- Your milk isn't good enough

  This is all extremely unlikely and counterproductive.

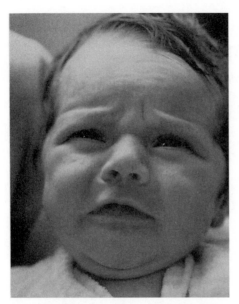

This baby looks worried. Part of parenting is learning to read your baby's signals—different facial expressions mean different things.

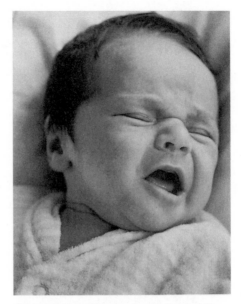

Because this baby is turning his head to the side, as if looking for the breast, it is likely to mean "I am hungry." If she has already fed well, then it could mean "I am tired and want to sleep." Over time you will be able to read his signals.

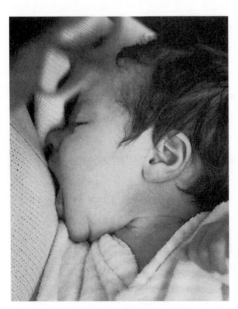

This probably means, "I'm hungry!"

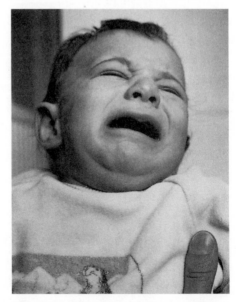

This could mean "I'm tired!", "I'm uncomfortable!", "I hurt!", or "I don't know what's wrong!"

How to Tell if There Are Problems: A List of Signs and Symptoms

Here is a list of signs and symptoms you may have if you have a problem with breastfeeding. Note that some symptoms can have more than one possible cause. It is likely that you have a breastfeeding problem if:

Your nipples are

- Sore during and just after feeding (see pages 120-125)
- Squashed and flattened just after feeding (see pages 120-121)
- Bleeding during and after feeding (see pages 120-121)
- Red and painful between feeds as well as during feeding (see pages 120-125)

Your breasts are

- Swollen (see pages 116)
- Painful all over a lot of the time (see pages 116)
- Painful only in some areas (see pages 117-120)
- Flushed (see pages 117-120)
- Lumpy (see pages 117-120)
- Not usually soft and feeling comfortable after feeding (see pages 117-118)

Your baby

- Is restless during feeding (see pages 125-129, 130-136)
- Pulls away from your breast during feeding and looks upset or cries strongly (see pages 125-129)
- Has difficulty staying attached to your breast, even with lots of help with positioning (pages 122-123)
- Never finishes feeding spontaneously (does not let go of your breast on her own) (see pages 125-129)
- Usually has long feeds (routinely longer than an hour) (see pages 125-129)
- Feeds very frequently (every one and a half hours or less from the beginning of one feed to the beginning of the next) both day and night (see pages 125-129)
- Frequently cries immediately after feeds (see pages 125-129, 130-136)
- Cries inconsolably for long periods (see pages 130-136)

- Does not pass the normal greenish black stool (meconium) in the first few days after birth (see pages 120-122, 136-138)

- Does not develop a breast milk stool (see pages 120-122, 136-138) by the end of the first week after birth

- Has a liquid stool, usually greenish in color (see pages 128-129)

- Never feeds deeply and rhythmically (see pages 120-122)

- Is not gaining weight (see pages 125-129)

- Chokes, possets, or spits up because she is overwhelmed by the amount of milk she is getting (see pages 128-129)

- Remains jaundiced (yellowish skin color) one to two weeks after birth (see pages 136-138)

Problems with Milk Flow: Description, Causes, Prevention, and Solutions

It is important that your milk be removed regularly from your breast, either by feeding your baby or by expression. This is to help maintain your supply and keep the milk moving.

Problems with milk flow may occur because:

- Your baby is not positioned well and therefore cannot milk the breast properly.

- Your milk supply exceeds your baby's demand. (This is often true for a few days after birth; milk is plentiful but your baby may not yet be feeding efficiently.)

- You may not be able to feed your baby as often as you need. Sometimes this happens if you leave the baby longer than usual between feedings.

If you are having a problem with milk flow, ask yourself:

1. Have I had too many visitors who want to play with the baby?

2. Are there people around who make me feel uncomfortable feeding in their presence?

3. Did I cut down on breastfeeding suddenly, for any reason?

4. Is there an obstruction to milk flow? (This may be caused by clothing, usually a bra or dress that is too tight, or by your fingers pressed into the breast when feeding.)

Problems with milk flow may lead to complications, as discussed here.

Painful, Swollen Breasts (Engorgement)

Having painfully swollen breasts (commonly known as engorgement) is usually a sign that milk is not flowing effectively from the breast. It frequently happens between the second and fourth days after birth, and indicates that your baby and your breasts are out of balance with each other. It can also happen if:

- Your baby is not positioned well enough to drain the breast efficiently

- Your baby is not able to feed frequently

- Your baby is not feeding for long enough

- If you are expressing, it may indicate you are not draining the breast efficiently

  As a result:

- Milk builds up in the breast

- This causes a slowdown of the blood and lymph supply

- You get painful, swollen breasts from too much milk, blood and fluid in the tissues (edema)

To fix engorgement breastfeed well and often! Check that your positioning is right (see pages 33-42), or ask someone skilled for help. If you are expressing, ask for help to check your technique.

Let your baby feed as often as she wants, and for as long as she wants. Do remember to let her feed until she is finished on the first side. She may not want the other side, but she'll take it at the next feed.

You may need to express a little milk before you start to feed: your breasts may be so full, she cannot get a good mouthful of your breast.

For quick relief from pressure and pain, express a small amount of milk in between feeds. Try doing this in a warm bath or a shower, or after placing warm, wet cloths on the breasts.

You may be told by some helpers or friends not to express your milk. It is a common misunderstanding that expression makes engorgement worse. *This is not true.* Gentle expression helps relieve the pain. Once you feed your baby well and express just enough to relieve the pain, the problem will resolve itself in a day or two.

If the pain is severe, and expressing a bit of milk does not relieve it adequately, you may want to take some pain relief for a very short time (usually less than one day).

Red, Inflamed Breasts (Mastitis)

If any part of your breast becomes red, inflamed, or hot to the touch, you have mastitis. Mastitis is caused principally by problems with milk flow. It may or may not be infected.

Mastitis is more likely to occur when:

- You have not fed your baby as often as usual

- Your baby is not positioned well

You may have been told to use a finger to hold your breast out of your baby's way. If you have been doing this, pressure from your finger on the soft breast tissue may have blocked milk flow from that area and caused the mastitis. If your baby is well positioned, there is no need to use your finger to keep your baby's nose clear. Some mothers find that breastfeeding is easier on one side than the other. Mastitis often occurs on the side that women find more awkward.

Mastitis commonly occurs when unusual events interrupt the normal pattern of feeding. Examples are:

- Going back to work for the first time

- Going out to an exciting event, such as a party

- Disrupting your normal feeding pattern because of travel

You may spend time organizing an event (such as your baby's christening or naming day) and looking after your visitors or houseguests so you do not feed your baby as often as she needs, and mastitis may result.

Mastitis may also occur if your clothing restricts the flow of milk and blood: for example, a bra that is too tight. You should choose your clothing with care.

How will you know if you are developing mastitis?

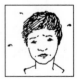

1. Part of your breast may feel painful, look red, and be hot to the touch.

2. You may feel hot all over.

3. You may have chills and shivers.

4. You may feel like you are getting flu.

Don't wait to see what happens. **Start treatment immediately so that it does not get worse.** The best possible treatment is:

1. **Feed your baby as often,** and for as long as she wants. This will keep your breast milk flowing, which is the root of the problem. Gently massage any lumpy or blocked areas while your baby feeds.

2. **Be especially careful with positioning.** Find someone to help you check positioning if you can, so that all of the breast are drained adequately.

3. **Try expressing milk.** Some women find that expressing milk as well as breastfeeding helps to resolve the problem. But if you do this, avoid bruising your breast by too much handling.

4. **Take care of yourself (and also ask others to care for you)** as if you had flu. Get lots of rest. Drink a lot of fluids.

You may find it helpful to take your baby to bed with you, so that you can feed the baby often and rest at the same time.

Do not stop breastfeeding. This will make the problem worse.

Try to feed so that the part of the breast that is inflamed is drained well by your baby. This may mean that you have to feed with the baby in a different position from usual: for example, if you usually feed with the baby tucked in close to your front, then try to feed with her tucked under your arm.

If the redness and pain do not start to resolve themselves within six to eight hours after you start treatment, then *contact a doctor.* Sometimes mastitis is caused by an infection, and if it is left to develop, a breast abscess may form (see page 119). This should never be allowed to happen. You may need an antibiotic. This will almost certainly help resolve the mastitis, but it may cause thrush in you or your baby (see pages 123-124) and should be used only when essential. Remember to complete any course of an antibiotic that you start; don't take it only until the symptoms disappear.

Blocked Ducts

Blocked ducts occur when the breast milk is not flowing well. You may feel a lumpiness anywhere in your breast, and it may or may not be painful.

This is an indication that positioning needs to be improved. Be careful to get it right at *every* feed (see page 35). You may find it helpful to try out some different positions. For example,

- If you usually feed sitting up, try lying down.

- If you normally feed with your baby under your arm, bring her around so that she is tucked into your front.

- You might also want to start with the side that has the lump for a feed or two, so that your baby feeds more vigorously on that side. Gently stroke the lump toward the nipple as you feed.

- Supporting the breast from underneath may help to promote better drainage.

White Spots

You may see small white spots developing on the tips of your nipples. These can be due to thrush (see pages 123-124), or they can show that the openings of the milk ducks onto your nipples are blocked with an accumulation of milk solids. Very occasionally, a thin layer of skin may grow over one of the openings on the nipple, looking like a tiny, milk-filled blister. If this is the case, and it does not get better with feeding and expression, you might like to try puncturing the skin with a sterile needle. You may want to ask for help from a health worker.

Treatment is similar to that for a blocked duct:

- Be careful with positioning, and try out some new positions.

- Gentle hand expression may also help; gently squeeze behind the spot; it should pop out and free the duct. Have a warm bath or shower first, or bathe your breast in warm water.

Do not persist in expression if it is painful; instead, feed your baby well and as often as she wants, and let her do the work for you. Good feeding will remove the blockage.

Breast Abscess

Warning: A breast abscess is a problem that needs medical attention immediately.

This is a *very* rare problem and is one that should never happen. It usually occurs if mastitis has not been treated, and it is the main reason why any episode of mastitis should be treated quickly and effectively. It may also result from infection entering the breast due to nipple damage. This is a good reason to treat the damage quickly.

If nipple damage does not heal, then the area around the nipple may become infected. If mastitis does not resolve itself, then the red, inflamed area may become infected.

In both cases you will find that the affected area becomes very painful and swollen, and you will feel quite ill (as if you have a bad attack of flu). You will have a fever. You may also find that you are losing some pus from your nipple. Pus is a good thing, as it helps the abscess to drain (but don't be tempted to squeeze it out).

Go to your doctor, who will start you on antibiotics. The abscess will probably need to be drained surgically. This may be done either by incision or by a needle (aspiration).

Do make sure you continue to feed your baby as often and as well as you can at this time. If you do not, then the problem may get worse. Remember that the cause in the first place was that milk was not being drained well from the breast. Even if you are losing pus from your nipple, you can still feed the baby; the pus will not harm her. If you do not want to do this, however, you can express your milk for a day or two, while you continue to feed from the other breast. If it is too painful to express, then breastfeeding your baby is usually the least painful way of moving milk. Although the wound may drain some pus and milk for a while, you can continue to feed or express.

It is very important that you do not wean suddenly at this time, as that would make the problem worst. If you have to go into the hospital for treatment, arrange for the baby to go in with you. If this is not possible, then make arrangements to express your milk regularly. If you have a surgical incision, you will need help to express your milk without interfering of the healing of the incision.

Problems that Cause Sore Nipples: Description, Causes, Prevention, and Solutions

Faulty Technique and Positioning

If your baby is not positioned well at your breast, a number of problems can result. These may occur in the early days as you learn about positioning. They can also occur later, perhaps because you are distracted and not as careful as usual at one or two feeds.

The most common problem that women develop with breastfeeding, especially in the first few days after birth, is sore nipples. *Sore nipples are not inevitable, and they should not occur.* It is almost always a sign that something is wrong with the way the baby is on the breast, and incorrect positioning will cause nipple damage. You may be able to see this damage as a crack in the nipple's surface or as bleeding. Sometimes the whole nipple becomes red. Perhaps you will not see any damage. But if it is sore, you can be sure that harm is being done. The soreness can usually be corrected by solving the positioning problem.

 Prevention is better than cure.

Some people will tell you that sore nipples are common, and that you should ignore them. *This is not true.* Pain is usually nature's way of indicating that something is wrong, and this is certainly the case with sore nipples.

The main cure for sore nipples is simple: get the positioning right. Read pages 35-37. Look carefully at the diagram and picture on pages 58-59. See how easy it is for your nipple to be damaged if your baby does not grasp enough breast when he takes the nipple. The strong suction that babies can exert will quickly flatten and damage a nipple that is in the wrong place.

Remember that both you and your baby must learn about and practice positioning. It doesn't always come easily. The baby cannot help you get it right: he has a reflex that encourages him to suck strongly on *whatever* is offered to him. You need to be very careful about reaching him to take the best mouthful of breast possible.

Do not let your baby stay on the breast if feeding makes your nipples sore. Take him off and try again, even if you have to take him off and put him on three or four or more times. It is important to keep trying until you get it right.

Take the time that you need to do this. It will be easier if you can find a skilled helper. If not, then ask your partner or a friend to give you moral support while you use the pictures on page 55 to get it right.

Even if your nipples are very sore, it will not help to stop feeding and rest them. It will also not help to use nipple shields to protect them. Resting your nipples or using nipple shields simply postpones solving the problem.

One you start to breastfeed again, your nipples will get sore again if you have not removed the cause. You may also complicate the problem by developing engorgement because you are not draining your breasts, and engorgement makes it even harder for the baby to get a good mouthful of your breast. Another complication can be that your milk supply is reduced because you don't have the regular stimulation of feeding.

Creams and lotions will not help either; some women find that they actually make the problem worse. Sensitive nipple skin may react easily to creams and lotions, and you may develop a skin problem (dermatitis) (see page 124).

If you want to put anything on your nipples, then put breast milk on them. It is high in fat and fights infection. It has no side effects and it's free. Express a few drops at the end of a feed and spread it on your nipples.

Sore nipples heal very fast once positioning is right. Sometimes after only one or two good feeds, damaged nipples are almost completely better. They should certainly be better within a day or two.

A note on babies vomiting blood: Some babies bring up a small amount of fresh blood mixed with milk after a feed. Others vomit what looks like a large amount of blood. *By far the commonest cause in both cases is breastfeeding from a damaged nipple.* This will not harm your baby, but you will be harmed if you do not resolve the problem. Talk to your health worker. Almost always your problem will be solved by curing your sore nipples.

Problems with the Baby's Tongue

A small number of women find that even though they are careful with positioning, they continue to have pain at some or most feeds. Ongoing pain which is not solved by careful positioning may be caused by the following:

- your baby's tongue is short and does not extend enough to grasp the breast well

- your baby has a tongue tie (the skin at the base of the tongue holds it so tightly that the tongue cannot extend properly)

Problems with the baby's tongue do not necessarily mean that feeding will be difficult. In spite of the fact that the baby's tongue cannot extend very far, some women find that their baby can draw enough of their breast in to feed well. But some women will experience pain while feeding, and this pain may be acute.

Understanding the problem is the first step. Women with ongoing acute pain who have tried hard to position the baby well are likely to feel that the problem is caused by their inability to get it right. Once you know the reason, and that it's not your fault, you can start to work out the solution.

First, check inside the baby's mouth. Can he extend his tongue over the edge of his lower gum? If not, is this because his tongue is short, or because the skin at the base of is tongue is tight? You will not need to put your fingers in the baby's mouth; when he is calm and alert, simply touch the baby's bottom lip. He will respond by opening his mouth and darting his tongue forward. Watch how far it extends; does it cover his lower gum? You might want to ask a health worker to check this with you.

If he has a short tongue, it will grow and become more flexible with time. This may take a week or two, or a month or two. Depending on how painful you find the feeds to be, you may need to express your milk and feed from a cup, spoon or bottle during this time. Do continue to give some feeds if you can; you will be able to feel the gradual improvement and help the baby to take the breast well. If you are careful with positioning every time you try to feed, you will find that the baby is able to take a good mouthful of breast and over time feeds will become more comfortable.

Some women find that supporting the breast from underneath throughout the feed helps, using their hand or a sling (see page 49).

If your baby has tongue tie, there may also be a gradual improvement over time. In some countries, doctors are happy to carry out a simple operation in which the thin skin at the base of the baby's tongue is nicked to release the restriction (frenotomy). This takes a second or two. It often does not need an anesthetic, and there is almost no blood loss. Babies can feed as soon as the procedure is carried out, which calms them and lets you feel the difference. In other countries, doctors do not wish to do this procedure. Perhaps this is because they are concerned that it may cause problems, or perhaps, in countries where bottle feeding has been common for years, doctors are no longer aware of the difficulties tongue tie can cause for breastfeeding mothers. If you do not want the procedure carried out, or it is not possible to have it carried out, the solution will be the same as outlined above for babies with short tongues. Express your milk, pay careful attention to positioning when you do try to put the baby to your breast, and wait for the baby to grow enough so that feeding becomes less painful.

Thrush, or Yeast Infection

Sore nipples are not always caused by positioning. Some women develop thrush (a yeast infection, also called candida) in their nipples. This can happen at any time while feeding: either when the baby is very young or when he is older. It can be caused by antibiotics. Some women are prone to vaginal thrush, and if so they may also develop thrush on the breasts.

Thrush, or yeast infection, on the breasts can cause:

- Itchy, irritable, slightly pink nipples and areolae. You may also see tiny white spots on your nipples.

- Red, exquisitely painful nipples and areolae that are sore both during and after a feed.

- Pain radiating up the breasts from the nipples, especially just after a breastfeed.

- Red sores on your baby's bottom, or white material (plaques) stuck to the inside of his mouth (oral thrush), or white spots on the back of his throat.

Thrush can happen after a period of trouble-free feeding. If you are prone to thrush, you should be especially careful while breastfeeding. It can be one side effect of using antibiotics for yourself or your baby, as it disturbs the normal balance of microorganisms in the body. Watch carefully for signs of thrush if you use antibiotics.

If you have thrush it is important to treat both yourself and your baby. It is easy to keep reinfecting each other if you do not. It is also important to treat it quickly, as it can be very painful for you (it is rarely painful for the baby). It can be treated efficiently and well.

Treatment of thrush is as follows:

- Ask your health worker for a prescription or medication to treat thrush. This should be an antifungal treatment (nystatin or miconazole are the generic names of two medications). You will need to treat both your nipples and your baby's mouth. You may also need to treat your vagina and your baby's bottom.

- Spread the antifungal cream on your nipples and your baby's bottom, and put the medication into your baby's mouth, using a cotton pad or dropper. Leave your baby's diaper off for a few hours, if you can, if he has a sore bottom.

The treatment should work in one to three days.

- If the infection is resistant, you or your baby may need to take oral treatment, which works on the whole body (systemic treatment). This is usually needed to treat radiating breast pain, which will take about a week to resolve itself.

Men can have thrush and show no symptoms. If the infection recurs after treatment, make sure all of you—baby, partner, and yourself—are treated the next time.

There is a sound theoretical basis for the use of a home remedy, bicarbonate of soda (common baking soda), to treat thrush both on the mother's nipples and in the baby's mouth. If you wish to try this, place 1 tsp. (5 ml) of baking soda in 1 cup (230 ml) of sterile water or water you have boiled for 20 minutes. If you put the solution in a jar with a tight lid, you can keep it with you and use it for as long as necessary. Each time you use it, shake it up and moisten a clean cloth or cotton swab. Use the solution both on your nipples and on the inside of your baby's mouth.

Dermatitis, or Irritation of the Skin

Some women develop an inflammation of the surface of the nipples, sometimes extending to the areolae, while breastfeeding. This can occur at any time. It is usually caused by reaction to something that you have put on your nipples, such as a cream or ointment. It can also be caused by contact with clothing or sensitivity to a soap or detergent you use to wash clothes.

Removing the cause of the irritation may be all that you need to do. Stop using the cream, keep only soft natural fabrics next to your nipples, change your detergent. Use air to dry your nipples after bathing.

In the very rare cases where the irritation does not resolve itself, ask your doctor for a prescription for hydrocortisone cream, 0.5 percent. This should be applied very sparingly for only two or three days, and you should gradually reduce the number of times you apply it. Do not stop the treatment abruptly, because if you do the problem will recur.

Problems of Milk and Milk Supply: Description, Causes, Prevention, and Solutions

Not Enough Milk

Today, when there is so little confidence in breastfeeding in many cultures, almost all women wonder at some time whether they have enough milk for a baby. Some wonder because their babies do not gain weight as quickly as the charts say they should. Some women doubt their milk supply if their babies cry a lot. Others wonder if their babies want to feed more often or longer than "normal."

So it is not surprising that not having enough milk is often the reason given by women stopping breastfeeding or for supplementing their feedings. In fact, some studies have found that as many as 75 percent of the women who stop breastfeeding in Western cultures do so because they feel they do not have enough milk to feed a baby!

Only a tiny percentage of women (probably less than 1 percent) are truly not able to produce enough milk to feed their babies. After all, women's bodies sustained their babies' lives during pregnancy; why should their bodies become incapable of sustaining their babies' lives after birth?

It simply does not make sense that so many women would be incapable of making enough milk. If this were the case, the human race would not have survived all the years before artificial baby milks were invented. Instead, it is likely that when a baby does not receive enough milk it is for a reason that can be corrected. Insufficient milk is most likely to be problems with positioning or problems with milk flow, both correctable problems.

If your baby is not well positioned at the breast, then she will not be able to make enough milk to satisfy her hunger. And because the amount of milk your body makes depends on the amount of milk your baby takes (see pages 66-67), you will not make enough milk, because only a small amount is being taken from your breasts.

There is wisdom in the body. It tries to make only as much milk as is needed. That is why the quantity of breast milk can go up and down according to the baby's changing needs. It is also why, when supplements are given to babies, women's bodies respond by making less milk, as their babies take less from them.

Similarly, if a baby is not able to feed often enough, or for as long as she needs, then the woman will not make as much milk as her baby needs. So it is likely that women who have not had enough help with positioning their baby correctly, who have been taught to limit their feeding times, or who give supplementary bottles will no longer produce enough milk. The result is a dissatisfied, crying baby who does not gain weight well, even though she may be at the breast almost constantly. This baby may not wake for a feed or may fall asleep immediately after starting to feed because she is hungry and not getting the food she needs.

Insufficient milk is almost always a problem that can be treated. It is best if you start to treat it soon after you suspect a problem, rather than waiting until both you and the baby are tired and frustrated and you are anxious and your baby is hungry.

To treat the problem of not having enough milk:

1. **Check your position and that of your baby carefully.** For some women and their babies, even a small change in position matters. So check the photographs and drawings in this book carefully and compare them to the way your baby looks while on the breast. Don't forget to check your own body position too. Sometimes, when you are anxious, you might concentrate more on your baby, when the problem could actually be solved by moving yourself a bit more upright. This makes it easier for your baby to grasp a bit more of your breast in her mouth.

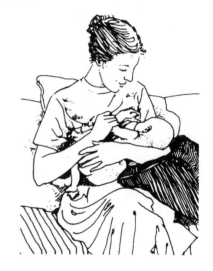

Some babies can feed well, and some mother can make plenty of milk, even if the positioning is not quite perfect. But there are some mothers and babies who seem to need it to be exactly right; these babies are often small babies, who tend to be sleepy and slow to suck. If they have exactly the right mouthful of breast tissue they do well, but if the positioning of either mother or baby does not look exactly right, then they tend not to respond and not suck well.

Getting the position exactly right is also important for some women who have large, soft breasts (see page 49 for what to do). It is really worth persevering to solve this problem. The most important things are patience, time, and an understanding of the ways to get positioning right.

3. **Encourage your baby to feed as often, and for as long, as possible.** This may be very often for the first two or three days after you start to treat the problem, because your baby will be hungry as if catching up, and it will take a day or two for your breasts to respond to the increased demands. If you can arrange to have help in the house, then do so; you may find it best to go to bed with your baby, and feed as often and for as long as you can for a couple of days. Make sure you are careful with positioning at each feed.

It is important to have confidence in your body: it will respond, but it will take a couple of days before you really see the results and probably one or two weeks before your breasts and your baby are really in balance.

Think carefully before giving supplements to your baby at this time. It is a difficult decision to make, because your baby is hungry; but supplements do make it harder to produce milk. On the other hand, if the problem of insufficient milk is long-standing, and there is concern that your baby is not gaining enough, then careful supervision by a skilled person is needed. The treatment is still as previously described, but there may be a need for ongoing supplementation for the baby too.

Too Much Milk! (Oversupply)

A very small number of women seem to have too much milk for their baby's needs. It is most common in the early days of breastfeeding, because the breasts have not settled down to producing only what that particular baby needs.

If it continues for a week or so, there are two causes: the baby not being well attached to the breast, or the baby being taken off one breast in order to make it feed on the second breast.

These are the symptoms of oversupply, and you are likely to have most or all of them:

- Your breasts normally get full and tender between feeds, even after some weeks of breastfeeding
- You leak milk to the point that your clothes are almost always wet
- Your baby pulls away from the breast during a feed, choking and spitting
- Your baby gets distressed while feeding, sometimes even at the beginning of a feed
- Your baby brings up more that one or two mouthfuls of milk after most feeds
- Your baby gains weight very fast
- Your baby had normal but plentiful stools

It is worth waiting a week or two to see if the problem resolves itself on its own.

If you have checked with your health worker and she agrees it is a case of oversupply, do not be tempted to take your baby off the first breast and put her on the other side just to relieve the fullness. All she will do is take the foremilk from both sides, without getting to the hindmilk from either, and the problem will continue! Instead, express just enough from the full side to feel comfortable.

If the problem persists, and the baby is well attached to the breast, it may be worth deliberately feeding from only one breast at each feed. In this way each breast will be stimulated only every second feed, and the milk supply will soon be reduced.

The best judge of the timing of each feed is your baby. Only your baby knows when she has had a good balance of foremilk and hindmilk, and when left to her own devices, she will always come off the breast herself in due time, provided she is feeding correctly.

Treatment of this problem is simple:

• Check to be sure positioning is correct

• Let your baby feed for as long as she wants to on each breast

See pages 70-73 for more information.

Foremilk/Hindmilk Imbalance

Some of the women who have some of the symptoms listed above for oversupply will find their babies also have other symptoms. These will include:

• wanting to feed very frequently (more often that every 2 hours from the beginning of one feed to the beginning of the next, day and night)

• growing well, but not content

• pulling away from the breast

• being restless or fussy while feeding

• crying inconsolably either just after or between feeds

• wanting to feed for long periods (an hour or more at each feed)

• not coming off the breast spontaneously at the end of a feed

• having wet, sometimes frothy, yellow or green explosive stools

If these symptoms persist your baby may stop growing well.

These problems, which often occur in combination with each other, lead some women to believe that they do not have enough milk. It may even lead them to think that although they feel they have too much milk, their milk does not satisfy their baby because it is 'not good enough'. It is never the case that a mother's milk is not good enough for her baby.

The real problem is almost certainly that the baby gets too *much* foremilk at the beginning of the feed, and not enough hindmilk (see pages 70-73). So the baby gets enough quantity, but not a balanced quality. She gets too few calories, and she is hungry and wants to feed more often. She may also get too much sugar (lactose), which can cause distress and a loose yellow or green stool.

This problem may happen when the baby does not have enough breast in her mouth or when the mother restrict breastfeeds and takes her baby off the breast at a set time. It seems to occur most commonly in mothers with an abundant milk supply.

Examples of situations that might create a foremilk/hindmilk imbalance are:

1. Imagine that the baby is not well attached to the breast. She does not have enough of the breast in her mouth to be able to milk the breast well. If you have an abundant milk supply, she will get good amounts of foremilk, but will not be able to draw down the higher-fat hindmilk well enough. So she must satisfy her hunger by drinking larger amounts of foremilk.

2. Imagine that you have been told to take your baby off the first breast after five or ten minutes and put her on the second side. She may not have reached the hindmilk on the first side yet. She will still be hungry and will feed well on the second side, but will get a second helping of low-calorie foremilk, rather than the high-calorie hindmilk she needs. She will come off the second side, having taken a lot of milk, but without the right balance of foremilk and hindmilk. She may not have reached the hindmilk on the second side because she got too full.

   She will be hungry soon after feeding, in spite of the fact that she seems to have fed well. What she needs is calories! She will want to feed frequently and may not gain weight well, in spite of the fact that she is taking lots of milk.

3. In the mistaken believe that the problem is simply oversupply, you may be told to feed from only one breast at each feed. As a result, you let her finish the first side and then stop. But your baby may still be hungry, and need some foremilk from the second side. She may even need both the foremilk and the hindmilk from the second breast. She too will still be hungry and will want to feed often. She may not gain weight well, yet appear to be feeding well. This advice is wrong and unhelpful.

Babies Who Cry a Lot:
Causes, Prevention, and Remedies

One of the hardest problems for parents to deal with is a baby who cries a lot. Crying is your baby's only way of trying to communicate what he needs and wants. Crying indicates a need, which may be:

- Hunger

- Pain

- Emotional distress

- Physical discomfort

- Overstimulation (when we are exhausted, we are likely to feel like crying!)

Sometimes it is not possible to satisfy the need and pacify the baby, but it is always important to try to work out what the cause may be in case you can help.

Over time you will learn the difference between your baby crying because of hunger and crying because of other reasons. The learning is a matter of trial and error.

One of the problems that has arisen from the common use of the term *demand feeding* (a term we never use in this book) is the mistaken idea that a baby needs to feed every time he cries. In fact, babies have a number of reasons for crying, and feeding is not always the answer.

It is almost always possible to calm an older baby by putting him to the breast, but a newborn will usually feed well only if he is hungry. If he is not hungry, he may fuss at the breast and possibly cry even harder. It may be worth trying, but do not persist if he is not interested.

A Note on Babies Who Do Not Cry

The other problem with the term *demand feeding* is the mistaken idea that babies always cry when they are hungry. In fact, some babies do not cry when hungry. If you have a very quiet, sleepy baby, who is not interested in breastfeeding you will have to make sure he feeds as often as he needs. Unusual quietness or sleepiness happens most often in the first few days after birth if:

- Your baby is small or sick

- You had medication during labor or an anesthetic (drugs affect the baby longer than they affect you)

- Your baby is jaundiced

It is unlikely that the sleepiness and disinterest in breastfeeding will persist after the first week, but it is important in these circumstances to feed your baby often, with no longer than five or six hours between each feed.

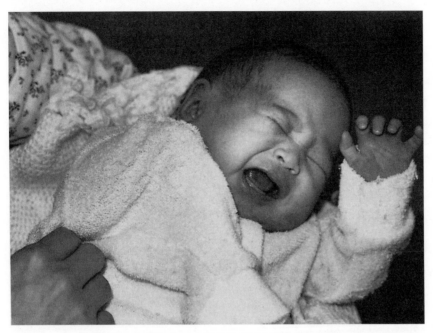

Many parents find the most difficult part of parenting to be coping with a young baby who cries and cries and cannot be consoled. Babies communicate many things through crying; it is not always easy to find the cause. People often call this kind of crying colic.

Working Out Why Your Baby Is Crying, and What to Do About It

The first question to ask yourself is, *When* does my baby cry? If it happens immediately after a good feed, then he is unlikely to be crying from hunger. He may be crying because of wind or gas or the discomfort that comes before passing a large bowel movement. Or it may be that in the early days after birth, as he adjusts to the feeling of a full stomach, he feels uncomfortable for a short while after he feeds.

If any of these are the reasons for crying, then one or more of these treatments may be useful:

- Burp your baby (just hold him in an upright position and the wind or gas should come up easily).

- Hold and comfort him.

- Check to see if his diaper or nappy needs changing.

- Cuddle him quietly. Try different positions: upright or on his tummy. Always tuck him in close to you. A baby sling that holds him close to you might help.

- Swaddle him in a wrap or blanket. Tuck his arms across his chest and wrap him firmly, so he is warm and secure.

Sometimes playing calming music, or walking the baby in rhythm to this helps. Your baby may respond to being cuddled and stroked in a warm bath with you. (Before getting in the bath with the baby, make sure it is not too hot for him: test the water on the inside of your wrist.) Or he may respond positively to gentle humming in his ear, especially a low note. (Try humming a single note for a moment or two.)

Sometimes a crying baby just will not stop, no matter what you do. Just let him cry but stay with him, cuddle him, and don't let him feel abandoned. Sometimes this will be hard to do; you may feel frightened of him or angry with him. If this happens, then ask for help with your baby from another caring adult.

A baby who cries after a feed and does not respond to your efforts may be indicating that there is a problem with the timing of the feed. This may happen if you have been advised to take the baby off the breast after a fixed period of time. This can cause two problems:

1. He may not have had enough milk, and may need to be left on the breast longer.

2. He may not have had enough hindmilk, which he should get toward the end of the feed.

Although your baby does not need much hindmilk, it is important that he get the high-calorie hindmilk as well as large quantities of the foremilk. This is explained on pages 66-67.

The solution to these problems is imply to leave your baby on the breast for as long as he wants (see page 67). If he takes a long time at each feed (regularly taking more than fifty to sixty minutes), then check the positioning (see pages 33-42), because it is possible that he is not feeding as efficiently as he could.

Sometimes a baby who has had repeated difficult experiences at the breast will cry in obvious distress when put to the breast. This baby is responding in the only way he knows how to the fact that he has learned that breastfeeding is frustrating.

This baby needs to learn that being close to the breast is pleasurable. He also needs to experience a good, satisfying feed. Imagine if every mealtime was painful for you. You would soon learn to dread mealtimes and not want to eat, and you would lose weight rapidly. The same is true for a baby.

It is important to prevent this problem if you can. This is another reason why it is so important for the baby to have a good experience at every single feed, right from the first feed: this way he will learn that feeding is pleasant and easy.

Remember to cuddle and calm your baby before you try to feed. Otherwise he learns to associate your breast with distress.

If this problem has developed, then remember that two things are important:

1. Both you and your baby must learn to associate contact with the breast with warmth and pleasure rather than pain and frustration.

2. Your baby needs to feed well and continue to gain weight.

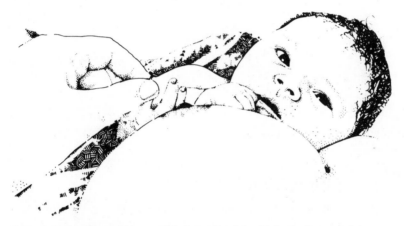

If your baby has learned to associate breastfeeding with frustration and distress, take time to be with him without trying to feed. Lots of skin to skin cuddles to help him and you associate your breast with comfort rather than distress.

Ways of solving this problem include the following:

- When you and your baby are both calm, take time to be with him. When possible, lie down with him next to you, with skin-to-skin contact. Keep him well cuddled into your breast, so that he can see, feel, and smell it. Do not try to feed him if he is not interested. Just cuddle and stroke him.

- Make sure he has enough food. If it is impossible for him to feed well at the breast, then you need to express your milk to keep your supply going (see pages 86-90) and feed this milk to your baby by spoon, cup, or bottle (see pictures of how to feed using these methods, page 102).

- Once he has learned that the breast is a comforting and pleasurable place to be, and his hunger is satisfied, you can bring him back to the breast. This should take only a few hours and a couple of good feeds. It is usually best to do this when he is not very hungry. If you can, have some help available for positioning him. Hold him close to you, encourage him to open his mouth wide, and move him onto the breast as shown on pages 59-60. Some people find it helps to express some milk into the baby's mouth before he goes on; the taste excites him. Don't persist if he cries; just cuddle and stroke him until he settles down, and then try again.

Remember to take a few slow, calming breaths and do anything else that calms you before attempting to feed. Soothing music can help put you in a relaxed mental state. Often it takes only one good feed for you and your baby to feel quite differently about breastfeeding.

If your baby will not be comforted and cries hard for long periods with no apparent cause, don't despair. It is likely he would behave the same way if you put him on a bottle. Find support for yourself and keep looking for the source of the crying. Others may have helpful suggestions. At the worst, and if nothing else helps, then sit tight until he is three or four months old, at which time this type of crying (sometimes called colic) often stops.

Food Sensitivity (Allergy/Intolerance)

Sometimes a baby cannot be comforted easily after a feed or throughout the day because he has developed a sensitivity to food that you are eating. Traces of this food pass through the breast milk to the baby. A baby can be allergic to any food. Some people will advise you not to eat certain foods when breastfeeding. But, in fact, food sensitivity differs from one mother and baby to another. It is impossible to generalize from someone else's experience.

If you are concerned that your baby may have food sensitivities, then ask yourself the following questions:

- Does my baby cry inconsolably for long periods?

- Does my baby find it difficult to settle down and sleep for any length of time and look anxious and unhappy much of the time?

- Does my baby have any other signs of sensitivity, such as rashes, dry, rough skin, or eczema, or a raw-looking bottom after passing a stool?

- Has my baby been given any formula or other food or drink that might have contained something to which he is sensitive?

- Have I tried to investigate all of the other possible causes of this crying?

If you find you cannot help your baby's crying by any of the ways already described in this section, then explore three other areas:

1. Do you smoke?

2. Do you drink coffee or other beverages with caffeine?

3. What do you eat?

Recent evidence shows that women who breastfeed and smoke are more likely to have babies with inconsolable crying, or colic. This happens because substances from smoking are passed into the breast milk. It may be worth the effort to stop smoking to have a settled baby. Don't expect the crying to stop immediately; it takes a few days or more to remove the toxins from your body.

A high intake of caffeine by breastfeeding women seems to be linked with excessive crying of their babies. Monitor the amount of coffee and tea you drink, and remember that many soft drinks contain caffeine too. Try cutting down on these beverages and drink water, fruit juice, or herbal tea instead. Many soft drinks now have caffeine-free versions. Again, you are unlikely to see immediate changes in the amount your baby cries when you stop or cut down your caffeine intake. It may take a few days for the caffeine to stop affecting your baby.

Next take a careful look at your diet. It is best to do this with skilled help, as any diet is complex. To start looking at your diet, ask yourself the following questions:

- Does anyone in my family or my partner's family have allergies?

- Was I bottle fed in infancy and given solids very early?

- What foods have I eaten in the past two days? (It takes varying amounts of time for food to enter your bloodstream and then your milk.)

  If you keep a diary of foods eaten for the two days prior to when your baby has a bad bout of crying, it may be obvious what food to suspect.

- Am I eating any food that I do not really like, but that I think is good for the baby?

  An aversion to a certain food is often a good indication that your body has a problem with that food. If that is the case, it is not wise to force yourself to eat it. It is not uncommon for women who are pregnant or breastfeeding to drink extra cow's milk, up to a pint or two a day. They may do this even when they do not like milk and do not normally drink it because they believe it is good for their growing baby. This can then cause problems for the baby, who may be sensitive to cow's milk as a result of the mother's sensitivity.

The mother herself may have symptoms that worsen; for example, headaches (including migraine headaches) or skin symptoms.

- Am I eating particular foods for which I have regular cravings?

  You may, conversely, develop a *craving* for a food to which you are allergic, such as eggs, peanuts, or chocolate. If your body is not handling a certain food well, your baby may become sensitized to it.

If you suspect a specific food sensitivity, try eliminating the most likely food for a week or two. You should notice a difference in your baby by then. Sometimes the baby's behavior may get worse for a day or two before it gets better. This is because of withdrawal; the baby will then improve after a week or so.

If you elect to cut out foods you suspect may be a problem, cut out only one kind of food at a time. If, for example, you suspect that you are sensitive to cow's milk or eggs, then cutting out both of these might solve the sensitivity problem, but it will not tell you which food is causing that problem. Cutting out a number of foods also makes it harder to eat a balanced diet. The more food you eliminate, the more difficult it is to balance your diet.

Other Problems: Description, Causes, Prevention, and Solutions

Jaundice

Jaundice occurs when the baby's body finds it hard to break down, or get rid of, a substance called bilirubin. Bilirubin is yellow and this is why babies look yellow when they are jaundiced. They have too much bilirubin in the bloodstream. The higher the level of bilirubin in the blood, the more yellow the baby looks.

The aim in treating any form of jaundice is to get the bilirubin level down to a normal level.

Jaundice is common and sometimes reaches higher levels in breastfed babies. A breastfed baby often will take longer to get rid of the greenish black stool (meconium) that is in the newborn's guts than a bottle fed baby will.

If breastfeeding is limited in frequency or duration, or if the baby is not well positioned, then he will not take as much colostrum or milk as he needs, and so delay passing his meconium.

Meconium is rich in bilirubin, and it seems to get reabsorbed into a baby's body if he does not pass it quickly. Colostrum, which your breasts produce in the first day or two after birth, has a good laxative action and will help your baby to pass stools at the right rate for a breastfed baby.

It is likely that jaundice is actually *caused* by some of the inaccurate feeding advice that has been given for so long, especially the advice that has limited the amount of colostrum and breast milk that babies have had in the first few days.

To prevent and to treat jaundice, which is usually at its peak on the first, third, or fourth day after birth, you baby needs to:

1. Breastfeed soon after birth,

2. Breastfeed well, and

3. Breastfeed whenever he wants right from the first feed.

Often it is recommended that a baby be given extra water or glucose to help with jaundice. This is not useful and is likely to slow down the establishment of your own milk supply (see pages 66-67). Breastfeeding well is often all that is needed to eliminate the jaundice. Water or glucose solution may actually increase the problem of jaundice, because they do not contain the protein that your baby needs. Giving these fluids also reduces the stimulus you need for your baby to make milk.

Other people may suggest that you wake and feed your baby every three hours. This may not help. Babies feed well only when hungry. You should concentrate on making every feeding as effective as possible, and feeding when, and for as long as, your baby wants. If your baby is sleepy (as is common with jaundiced babies), you may need to wake him. But do not try to force him to feed from your breast. If he will not, express your milk and encourage him to take this breast milk by cup, spoon, or bottle.

Often, having one or two really good breastfeeds will quickly improve the jaundice.

A health worker may suggest phototherapy (light treatment) for your baby if the bilirubin level is high. Ask if it is really needed, as it is sometimes prescribed for even mild jaundice. In suitable climates some mothers choose to sit in the sun to breastfeed to expose the baby to the benefits of sunlight, rather than phototherapy light. *If you do this, take care to avoid sunburn.* If your baby is put under a bilirubin light, then be especially careful with feeding. Babies can get dehydrated as a result of phototherapy (they get diarrhea). This is a case where extra water might be necessary to treat the dehydration, especially if the phototherapy is continuous. If so, express milk in addition to breastfeeding, to keep up your supply. Breastfeed as often as you can.

Jaundice can also occur if:

- Your baby was born prematurely
- Your baby is bruised, perhaps as a result of a difficult delivery
- Your baby has an infection
- Your baby may have a blockage of the bile duct (biliary atresia)

In any of these cases your baby should be cared for by a pediatrician. In all cases the best thing you can do is give your baby our own breast milk, either directly from your breast or after expressing it.

Remember that it is important to maintain your milk supply and keep your milk flowing. If you cannot breastfeed directly, express your milk. See pages 86-90.

 Jaundice should never result in problems with breastfeeding. Instead, breastfeeding is usually the best treatment!

The most uncommon case of jaundice is called breast milk jaundice. In this case the baby reacts to a substance in the mother's breast milk or the mother lacks a substance in her milk. As a result the baby becomes jaundiced. This will happen after the first week, not in the early days. *This type of jaundice usually stays at a level that is noticeable but not dangerous.* The level falls gradually throughout the next few weeks. Since the jaundice will disappear of its own accord, you do not need to do anything different—just continue to breastfeed.

Until the level starts to fall, it is important to have the jaundice monitored by a health worker.

Some people may advise you to stop breastfeeding. This is almost never necessary. If the jaundice level becomes very high, then interrupting breastfeeding for a day or two while you express milk and feed your baby alternative milk (either donated breast milk or artificial milk) will be helpful.

Blood in the Milk

In the early days of breastfeeding, some women find that they have blood in their breast milk. It can come from one or both breasts. There is no pain or nipple damage associated with this.

This seems to be the result of the extra growth of the ducts during pregnancy. It will resolve itself in the next few days. Most women never notice what is happening unless the baby vomits.

Just keep breastfeeding, as the blood will not harm the baby. His stool may be a darker color than normal, and if he vomits or spits up there may be dark flecks in the milk. Do not be alarmed.

If the blood persists for more than a week, then contact a health worker. It is possible, but highly unlikely, that the bleeding indicates a more serious problem.

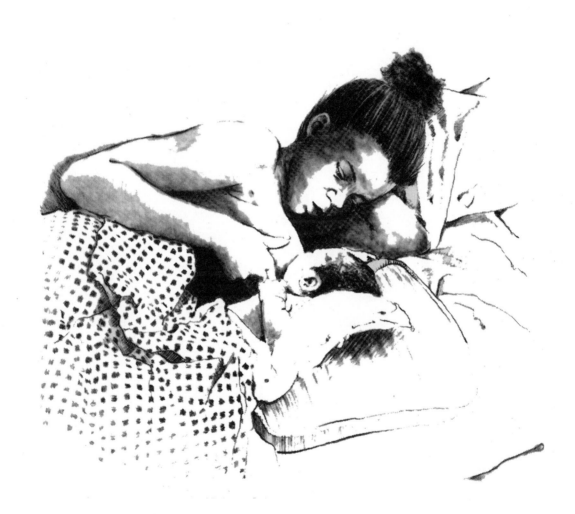

CHAPTER SIX

Why Women Have Problems with Breastfeeding

$\mathcal{A}$s we said before, most problems with breastfeeding can either be prevented or easily treated. Once women develop problems they often find that they are on their own. In many countries there is little support either from family (who often do not know the answers) or from health workers (who often do not know the answers either).

The fact that most breastfeeding problems are preventable or can be treated is not widely know by mothers or health workers. Why is this?

The reasons why so many women today have problems with breastfeeding are not entirely clear. But we do know some of the factors that have resulted in such problems for women and babies.

The Invention of Bottles and Artificial Milks

Until the early twentieth century, substitutes for breastfeeding were not readily available for all women. Mothers who were well off could hire women to breastfeed in their place (wet nurses). Other mothers gave substitutes of cow's or goat's milk, bread, and spices. The babies of these mothers died more often than those of mothers who breastfed.

Primitive commercial artificial formulas became available in the late nineteenth century. These were promoted by the manufacturers, and sometimes by the medical profession, as safe, even though they had never been tested on babies.

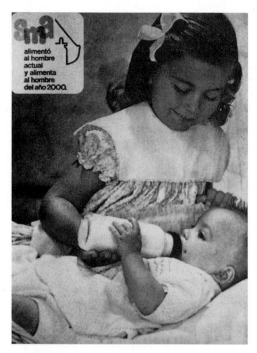

The invention of feeding bottles made artificial feeding more possible throughout the world. This Mexican poster shows how accepted bottle feeding has become in most countries.

Bottle feeding and breastfeeding are considered by many to be interchangeable and equal because bottle feeding is so heavily advertised and breastfeeding so misunderstood.

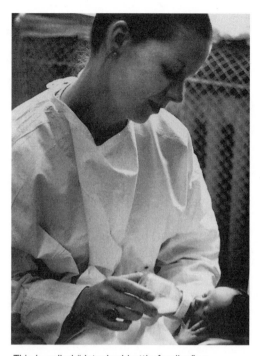

This is called "detached bottle feeding" because there is little body contact between the woman and the baby, as if the only important part of feeding were getting the food into the baby's stomach.

As the use of artificial substitutes for breast milk grew in Western culture, the knowledge about breastfeeding diminished. At the same time women started to work full days away from their babies, partly as a result of the World Wars, when women were needed to work in the factories, and partly because of the slowly increasing emancipation of women. No one really understood the impact this would have on child rearing.

Doctors then began to pay increasing attention to childbirth, and the results were mostly far from helpful. The advice written for mothers and caregivers by the new breed of infant feeding "experts" shows just how misguided much of this medical advice was. For example, breastfeeding mothers were taught to limit every breastfeed both in frequency and duration. Supplemental bottle feeding became widespread, probably because babies were left hungry after inadequate breastfeeds.

Modern Interventions in Birth and Infant Care

In the early 1900s widespread changes began to be introduced into the care of women at birth. Interventions in childbirth, many of them unnecessary, became routine. Gradually the hospital became the normal environment for birth. Interventions that were necessary in a few special situations quickly became the norm. Routine interventions included:

- Separating mothers and babies immediately after birth

- Placing healthy newborn babies in separate nurseries for observation

- Limiting the close contact between mothers and babies

- Scheduling and limiting breastfeeding

- Introducing bottles of artificial milk or sugar water to all breastfed babies

- Not allowing breastfeeding at night

- Teaching mothers to take the baby off the breast when the baby was judged to have had enough, usually after a specified time

- Encouraging the continued separation of mothers and babies at home, by advising parents to sleep in rooms separate from their babies' rooms right from birth

- Warning parents that picking babies up and cuddling them between feeds would spoil them

Bottles, schedules, and the separation of mothers and babies are interventions in breastfeeding, in just the same way as inductions, the use of oxytocin in labor, and cesarean sections are interventions at birth.

Just like all interventions in birth, they may be appropriate for a few mothers and babies. But they all have harmful side effects that outweigh the benefits when routinely applied to the majority of mothers and babies. Because these interventions now happen so often, most people have come to accept them as normal, often not questioning their use.

A good example of an intervention in birth that most accept as normal is not permitting a woman to eat or drink in labor, instead using an intravenous (IV) drip, which is painful and restricts movement. This is similar to giving newborn babies bottles of sugar water (which has no nutritional value and actually causes hypoglycemia), rather than letting them breastfeed freely. It is easy to forget the harm that IVs and sugar water can do, and also to forget that women and babies need real nourishment in labor and afterward.

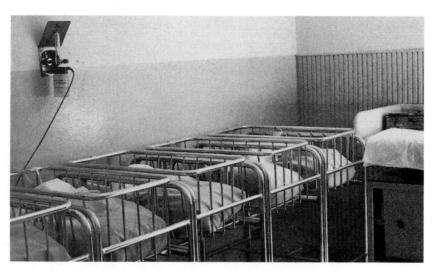

With routine intervention in normal birth has come the routine practice of separating babies from their mothers after birth. This is a hospital nursery in Italy, but it is still typical in many countries.

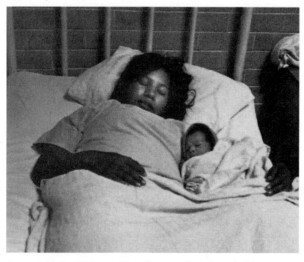

In most parts of the world mothers and newborn babies are kept together right from birth. This day-old Central American baby and her mother sleep together. If a mother prefers, she can place her baby in a little crib which is next to every mother's hospital bed.

The use of breast milk substitutes and of interventions in birth and breastfeeding has now spread from Western countries to virtually all countries. Their impact is felt all over the world, even in countries where breastfeeding was, until very recently, the norm. There are still a few societies where breastfeeding is the normal way of feeding a baby. We have a lot to learn from mothers who breastfeed their babies without interventions.

The Separation of Women and Babies from Each Other and from Social Contact

Mothers and babies are often separated not just after birth, but also after they go home. Putting babies to sleep in rooms separate from those of their parents is one form of separation. Mothers leaving the home for a full working day is another.

Choosing whether to go back to work is a dilemma many women face. In cultures in which home and work are separated and in which there is little social support form women who stay at home, women often must work outside the home and even outside the local community. Separation therefore lasts even longer than the working day. It is not unusual for a mother to travel an hour to and an hour from her work. Women need to work for many reasons: to earn money, for social contact, and to maintain promotion prospects in careers, which are shaped by the belief that workers (both women and men) should always put work first, never families or relationships.

In some countries (such as the United States and the United Kingdom) there is little support for women who wish to breastfeed and work outside the home. In other places, such as in Scandinavia, laws exist that enable women to work and have time and facilities to be with their babies and breastfeed during the work day.

A woman may choose to put her child in day care even if she does not work outside the home. In cultures in which the nuclear family is held as the ideal, it is sometimes hard for women to find enough adult company and support while caring for their own babies at home. Depression is now common among women in Western societies who stay at home to care for their babies and who become isolated from other adults. It is unhealthy to be separated from social support, especially when caring for young children. Some women assume that regular separation in this way means that they cannot continue to breastfeed. In fact they can, but they need support and facilities to do so, and these are not often available.

Working Away from Your Baby
(see also pages 10-11)

Until societies that separate women and their babies from other adults change, it will be necessary for some women to leave the home to go out to work while they have very young babies, and to put young babies in full-time day care, in spite of the problems this causes. Many women find the demands of both breastfeeding and working outside the home too difficult, so they stop breastfeeding. Others find it hard to maintain their milk supply when separated, and find they have to stop even though they do not want to. The best ways to prepare for breastfeeding when you work outside the home are:

- Get breastfeeding off to a good start

- Prevent problems

- Learn early how to express milk

The Acceptance of Bottles as the Normal Way of Feeding

Over the years most Western societies have become more comfortable with bottles than with breasts, partly because most people have been bottle fed, and partly because of discomfort with the exposure of breasts. In many countries there is little experience of successful breastfeeding. And in these countries bottle feeding is even seen as more normal than breastfeeding. Have you ever seen a breastfeeding mother on television? Have you ever seen breastfeeding mother and child dolls?

Think about how people often react with discomfort or criticism if a woman breastfeeds when outside her own home in Western countries. Breastfeeding is not an accepted part of modern life (although even up until World War II, it was common to see women in the United States and the United Kingdom breastfeeding in public). How would you feel if you were told you could not eat your dinner in public?

One of the most obvious symbols of the "normality" of bottle feeding is the common use of the bottle shape to indicate a feeding room in an airport or shopping center.

The acceptance of bottles is often unconscious. How many times have you heard people say things such as, "your breasts will be empty after feeding"?

Breasts are never empty; they make milk all the time. Only bottles are empty after feeding.

A common question mothers ask is, "How can I know how much milk my baby is getting?" You do not need to know the exact amount. The common use of bottles has accustomed people in Western countries to seeing how much babies drink. Thus they feel uncomfortable if they do not see it and cannot measure it.

Look carefully at the advertising for baby products and even at the birth congratulation cards that you get. Many of these include baby bottles.

Breastfeeding has been forced to meet the standards of bottle feeding. This is the opposite of the way it should be: artificial feeding should be required to meet the standards of breastfeeding.

A Lost Confidence in Breastfeeding

The common use of bottles and lack of experience with breastfeeding helps to explain why so many women have no confidence in their own bodies or their own babies when breastfeeding. For example, women have been told that giving feeds at certain times is the best way to feed. In fact, if they listened to their babies rather than this unhelpful advice, they would feed when the baby was hungry, not when the clock read a certain time.

Feeding by schedule can also harm the mother. Her breasts become engorged because they are not milked efficiently, and this causes pain and tissue damage. A mother responding to her own body would feed her baby more often and thus prevent or alleviate the problem.

It is easy to see, however, why people have lost confidence in breastfeeding. Because so many women, including the mothers of many of today's mothers, have bottle fed, there is little experience of normal breastfeeding in their communities. Women who have breastfed have often had problems because of lack of experience and support around them. Problems have become "normal."

The Problems for Health Workers

Remember that health workers are affected by cultural norms too. Whether they are nurses, midwives, doctors, lactation consultants, or nutritionists, they are not immune to social beliefs and experiences. Bottle feeding has been accepted for several generations in some Western countries. Textbooks and teaching for health workers are full of inaccurate advice. Much of the teaching of health workers in developing countries too is based on the experience and textbooks of Western medicine, in spite of the obvious lack of relevance of such information for most developing countries.

So health workers in most cultures find it hard to learn from experience. Books may still be unreliable sources of information. Many health workers are used to the common interventions, such as timing feeds and giving bottles, often not understanding that it can be otherwise.

For health workers to be confident in caring for you, they need to have experience working with confident breastfeeding women. Because this is rare, they depend on the misinformation they have learned.

It is striking that no modern health care system that we know of has a rational approach to infant feeding. Every system around the world contains at least some practices that are both irrational and actually damaging to breastfeeding. These include the routine interventions that we talked about earlier, and the fact that care is concentrated around the time of birth, with virtually no care for the mother and baby after birth in some countries, particularly in the United States.

In the United States, for example, where women give birth in hospitals and go home a day or two after birth, it is rare for women to receive *any* professional care at home at all. Where does a woman who needs skilled care after birth turn for help? In the United Kingdom, all women receive visits at home from their community midwife at least until the tenth day, and often for longer. They then have their health visitor to turn to for help. But where can they get help with housework?

It is understandably difficult for health workers who have little experience with breastfeeding, who have a fund of misinformation from textbooks, and who are often not around when problems occur, to offer women the help they need. No wonder the most common solution offered to mothers with problems is "Try bottle feeding."

Mixed Messages

Many health workers and laypeople do know that breastfeeding should be different from the way it has been. They have heard of many of the helpful practices. But they often have too little experience to truly have confidence in these practices. This often results in people giving mixed messages to women.

These people may be genuinely supportive of breastfeeding, but may say something like, "Yes, demand feeding is best for your baby; you'll find that he'll probably want to feed every three or four hours or so." Such a statement may leave you wondering what is wrong when your baby sleeps for two hours or five hours between feeds.

Another example is, "Let the baby feed as long as she wants; I will show you how to take her off the breast when she has had enough." You may then wonder how you can tell when she has had enough, instead of realizing that she will let you know by coming off the breast herself.

Some of the strongest of these mixed messages come from the companies that manufacture artificial substitutes for human breast milk. Advertisements for artificial milk often care a subtle (or sometimes obvious) message that artificial milk will be necessary when breastfeeding fails. That is why the World Health Organization has produced a code of practice for marketing of artificial milk. The message advertisements often give is that breastfeeding will not work, even if it is better than substitutes. We call this the breast-is-best-*but* approach.

Although artificial milk companies have attempted to produce substances that babies can tolerate and thrive on, and although their products are useful in some circumstances, the dissemination of mixed messages is damaging and inaccurate.

We all need to learn to trust in the ability of women's bodies to breastfeed successfully. Instead of thinking, breast is best *but* . . . people need to believe the truth: breast *is* best.

But it is only possible for people to truly have this confidence by either personally experiencing successful breastfeeding or by seeing others do it.

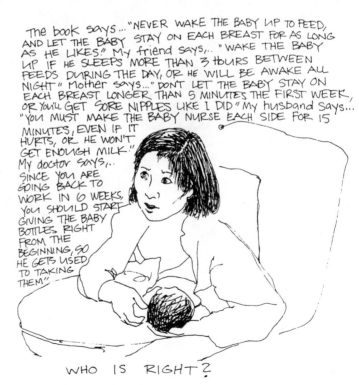

The book says... "NEVER WAKE THE BABY UP TO FEED, AND LET THE BABY STAY ON EACH BREAST FOR AS LONG AS HE LIKES." My friend says,.. "WAKE THE BABY UP IF HE SLEEPS MORE THAN 3 HOURS BETWEEN FEEDS DURING THE DAY, OR HE WILL BE AWAKE ALL NIGHT" Mother says..."DON'T LET THE BABY STAY ON EACH BREAST LONGER THAN 5 MINUTES THE FIRST WEEK, OR YOU'LL GET SORE NIPPLES LIKE I DID" My husband says... "YOU MUST MAKE THE BABY NURSE EACH SIDE FOR 15 MINUTES, EVEN IF IT HURTS, OR HE WON'T GET ENOUGH MILK." My doctor says,... SINCE YOU ARE GOING BACK TO WORK IN 6 WEEKS, YOU SHOULD START GIVING THE BABY BOTTLES RIGHT FROM THE BEGINNING, SO HE GETS USED TO TAKING THEM."

WHO IS RIGHT?

There is so much said about breastfeeding.

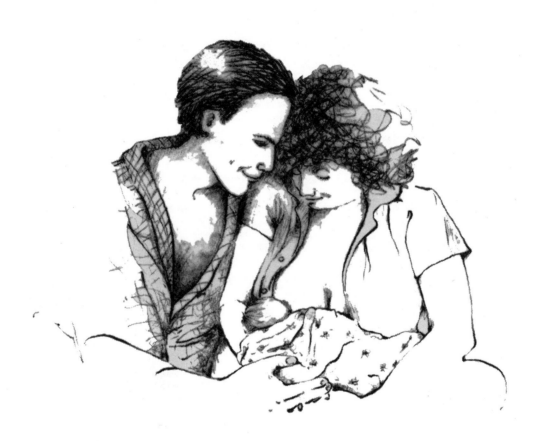

CHAPTER SEVEN

Things You Will Hear That Aren't True: Modern Myths

One of the problems you will have to cope with when you are breastfeeding, or planning to, is that many people will give you different, sometimes conflicting, advice and hints about feeding.

We explained some of the reasons for this (see pages 148-149). In addition, many people who have breastfed (or have heard of others who have), or who have cared for breastfeeding women, will give you hints based on their experience.

These hints may be invaluable. Or they may be quite wrong. This is not because these friends or helpers *intend* to mislead you; it is because of confusion and lack of knowledge about breastfeeding.

This may be true of much of the advice given by health workers, family, and friends.

You will have to battle to disentangle fact from fantasy! We hope the information that follows will help.

MYTH:

You must prepare your nipples in pregnancy to toughen them. If you do not they will become sore and damaged.

REALITY:

Nipples do not need to be tough, because in the right position they will not get damaged or be subjected to any friction inside the baby's mouth (see page 56). In fact, they need to be soft and pliable. No form of preparation has been shown to be of any help in avoiding damage.

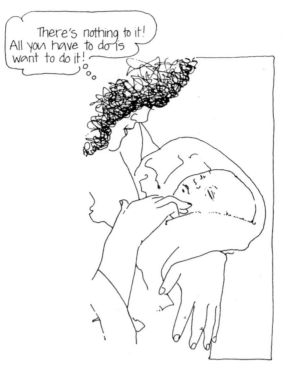

*Some women think it's so easy,
there's nothing to it.*

MYTH:

Women who have fair skin, red hair, or blue eyes will get sore nipples because
they have delicate, easily damaged skin.

REALITY:

No studies have ever shown that this is the case. These women, like all
women, simply need to have help with positioning, so that their nipples do not
get damaged (see pages 48-60).

MYTH:

You must feed your baby immediately after birth or breastfeeding will not
work.

REALITY:

This has never been shown to be the case. It has, however, been shown that in
cultures where immediate separation of mother and baby is the custom,

women who feed within two hours of birth go on to breastfeed longer than those who do not.

There are other cultures where women do not breastfeed for the first two or three days, and during that time the baby is given other fluids or food instead of breast milk. These women still breastfeed successfully.

There is no critical period, no crucial time beyond which breastfeeding will not work. The ideal time to breastfeed is within the first couple of hours after birth (see page 30), but don't panic if you can't or if your baby doesn't want to yet. Remember that even mothers who have adopted babies have been able to stimulate their milk supply.

MYTH:

You must time your baby's feeds, especially during the first few days, to prevent sore nipples.

REALITY:

Sore nipples are caused by bad positioning, not by the amount of time your baby spends at the breast. In fact, limiting feeding time actually *causes* problems for babies (see page 72).

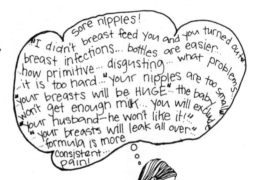

MYTH:

Babies must feed from both breasts at every feed, or the milk supply will not be stimulated well enough.

REALITY:

Babies should be allowed to decide what they want at each feed; any other method causes problems (see pages 72-73).

Some women think it's so difficult, they'll never be able to do it.

MYTH:

Babies must feed from only one breast at each feed; that is all they need.

REALITY:

This is the opposite of the preceding myth, but is equally popular. Again, babies should take what they need, not what rules and regulations decide is best (see page 72).

MYTH:

You must drink lots of fluids (up to twelve to fourteen glasses a day) or you won't make enough milk.

REALITY:

Studies show that this is not the case. All you need to do is drink when you are thirsty, rather than forcing yourself to drink more. Some women do get very thirsty, especially as they start to feed.

It is all right to drink whenever you want to. But be sure not to forget to drink; some women look after their babies more than themselves. If your urine is dark or strong-smelling, then you definitely need to drink more.

MYTH:

Most breastfed babies need bottles of water or artificial milk or they won't get enough fluid.

REALITY:

On the contrary, giving extra fluids to breastfed babies can reduce you milk supply and interfere with the special properties of breast milk. The colostrum and milk that you produce is all your baby needs, as long as you are feeding without problems and not limiting feeding times (see page 79).

MYTH:

The amount of milk a baby gets in a breastfeed is related to the length of that feed.

REALITY:

Studies have shown that some babies feed for four minutes to get the same amount as other babies take in twenty-five minutes. Each baby has her own rate of feeding, and each woman has her own rate of milk release. You and your baby will work out your own pattern, as long as the positioning is correct.

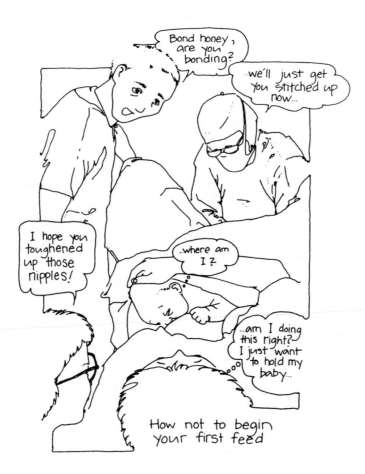

How not to begin your first feed.

MYTH:

To help her nipples to heal, a mother with sore or bleeding nipples should:
- Rest her nipples,
- Use a nipple shield,
- Use a cream, lotion, or spray, or
- Stop breastfeeding.

REALITY:

Unless the mother solves the *cause* of the problem (which is always either a positioning difficulty, an infection, or a skin reaction), then nothing will help. Some of the treatments just listed may actually make her problem worse. None will fix it, unless stopping breastfeeding can be called fixing it (see pages 120-125).

MYTH:

If you've fed before, you must know what you're doing.

REALITY:

Each baby is different and you need to learn each time how to breastfeed this baby. Having done it before helps, but it is not a guarantee. You can still have problems.

MYTH:

Flexible, or demand feeding, is harder on the mother.

REALITY:

Feeding your baby whenever she wants is the best thing to keep her contented. If you don't do this, then she will cry more than she needs, and this will disturb you and your whole family. This is *not* easier on the mother (see page 72).

MYTH:

If your baby feeds only from the breast, you will never get enough sleep at night.

REALITY:

It is true that breastfed babies wake in the night more often than bottle fed babies. And it is true that lack of sleep is the hardest problem for parents of young children. Unlike bottle feeding, however, once you and your baby are breastfeeding well, you do not have to be fully awake during a feed. Have your baby sleep near you, take him into bed when he cries (or have him sleep in the same bed with you and skip this step), feed lying on your side, and fall back to sleep (see page 36). Do not do this if you have consumed alcohol, and do not smoke if the baby is in bed with you (it's best never to smoke near the baby).

MYTH:

Women with engorged breasts should not express milk to relieve them.

REALITY:

Gentle expression of a little milk helps relieve engorgement and swelling (edema). It does *not* make it worse (see page 116).

MYTH:

Young babies always cry a lot, so you should leave your baby to cry.

REALITY:

A baby has all the feelings an adult has. She cries because she has a need. Crying only expresses pain or upset, nothing else. People comfort adults who cry. A baby cannot meet most of her own needs, and she needs us to take her crying seriously; she needs comfort too (see pages 131-134).

MYTH:

If you and your baby have serious breastfeeding problems, you won't be able to continue to breastfeed.

REALITY:

Most breastfeeding problems can be solved, even quite serious ones. Often the solution is simple and improvement happens quickly. The sooner you try to deal with your problem, the easier it is. Don't wait until it grows; deal with it now. See pages 114-115 for a listing of problems and solutions.

MYTH:

Orthodontic bottle or pacifier teats are the teats most similar to mothers' nipples.

REALITY:

Orthodontic teats are firm and hold a definite shape. They are not soft, responsive, or stretchy like mothers' nipples. We still do not know what shape of teat is least harmful to the development of the baby's face.

MYTH:

Your baby is sure to be feeding well if he has six to eight wet diapers or nappies a day.

REALITY:

In assessing your baby's health, you need to just several different factors, not just one. (For a listing, see page 83.)

MYTH:

You must begin to give solid foods when your baby is four months old or she will be nutritionally deprived.

REALITY:

Babies who are breastfeeding well can breastfeed without any other foot for at least six months, and some for longer. What matters is that they are content and continue to grow well.

MYTH:

You must stop breastfeeding by nine months, or you will never get the baby to stop.

REALITY:

This is not true. You and your baby can work out the best time for you both to cut down and then stop breastfeeding.

There are no hard and fast rules, and it will not harm your baby to continue for a long while, even after you have introduced other foods, if you both want to do so. In many cultures, children are normally breastfed for three or four years.

MYTH:

You must continue breastfeeding until the baby wants to stop, or you will harm her psychologically.

REALITY:

This myth is the opposite of the preceding myth. You feel pressure to continue longer than you may want to. You and your baby should work out together what is best for you both. As is true in any good relationship, you may both need to compromise.

MYTH:

You will spoil your baby if you give him what he wants whenever he wants it.

REALITY:

Responding to babies' needs is not the same as spoiling them. Babies need to be fed when they are hungry, to sleep when they are tired, to be cuddled when they feel lonely, and to be comforted when they are sad. This will result in contented babies, not little dictators. A contented baby is better equipped to handle the normal pains and frustrations that are part of being human than is a baby who is often frustrated and upset, but rarely comforted.

MYTH:

I don't care what anyone says, breastfeeding hurts. My health worker tells me this is normal, there is nothing I can do about it—I just have to put up with it if I want to continue breastfeeding.

REALITY:

If breastfeeding is going well, it should not hurt. Ongoing pain is a sign that something is wrong, and it should never be considered as "normal." In the early days, you may feel a sharp, sometimes painful sensation for the first few seconds of each feed, as your nipple and breast stretch or the baby starts to suck. This sensation should not last through the feed, and it should not continue for longer than the first week or two, as your nipples and breasts adjust to their new role.

If your nipples do get damaged, it will take a few days of careful positioning to fully heal. But you should feel a steady improvement through this time.

To prevent pain, and treat it after is has started, see pages 48-60.

MYTH:

I had to stop breastfeeding because my milk was too thin (or too rich).

REALITY:

Mothers make milk that is perfect for the needs of their own babies. Whatever your baby needs your body will produce. It is important not to follow unhelpful rules which restrict the time the baby has at each breast—your baby will let you know when she has had enough. The section on pages 70-73 will tell you more about milk composition. Your baby may cry and be unsettled for other reasons, which you will probably be able to solve by reading the section on "Getting the basics right." But the problem will not be caused by your milk being too thin, or too rich.

As your baby gets older, the appearance of your milk will change, so that at the start of a feed it may be almost transparent. Over time, it will look less and less like cow's milk—but it will still be just what your baby needs.

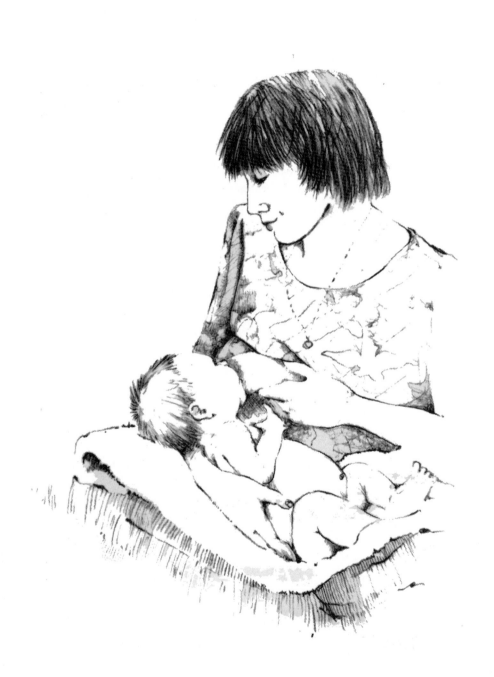

CHAPTER EIGHT

Women's Breastfeeding Stories: Case Studies

Every breastfeeding experience is different, and each mother faces different circumstances and challenges.

Some women have good support; others have none. Some have babies who feed well and easily from the start; others struggle for a while. Some produce lots of milk; others produce less. Some mothers are able to stay home full time while their babies are young; some must go back to work and leave their babies in the care of others for many hours a day.

Dealing with your own circumstances means that you need to understand the basic principles we outline in this book, and then adapt them to ourselves and your family. To show the wide variety of situations that women face when they breastfeed, we have included stories about women from different countries and ethnic backgrounds, showing how each woman dealt with her breastfeeding problem.

All of the women in these are people with whom we ourselves have worked. We've chosen problematic stories rather than easy ones to give you confidence in your own ability to work things out.

Please don't be put off by these stories, which are intended to help women with problems. Many women breastfeed easily, without any difficulty.

Becky's Story:

A Sleepy Baby Who Was Losing Weight

*J*ONATHAN was Becky's first baby, and she really wanted to breastfeed him. Her birth took place in a hospital. She had an epidural anesthetic during her labor, but went on to have a normal spontaneous delivery with a small episiotomy.

She kept Jonathan with her after the birth and fed him as soon as they were settled into bed together. A maternity nurse helped her with the first feed. Becky went home on the second day without anyone at the hospital watching her feed again or realizing that she had a problem. But Becky knew.

At home she got really discouraged when, after trying to put Jonathan on her breast as well as she could at each feed, he would cry fiercely and then get tired and lie there with her nipple in his mouth and fall back to sleep. He was a normal-sized baby at birth ($7 \frac{1}{2}$ pounds), but was down to 7 pounds after a week. Becky became even more frustrated when she found that when she gave him a bottle, he would drink thirstily and go to sleep contented. The swollen breasts that she had on the third and fourth days after birth made her problems even worse. She became so sore that she found it even harder to put her baby on her breast.

Becky asked for help from many people. By nine days after birth, she had seen five health workers. All tried to help; each gave different advice. She was told to wake Jonathan every two hours and try to feed him because he was still losing weight. She was also advised to give him three bottles of artificial milk a day.

Jonathan and his mother had never had even one good, pleasurable breastfeed. In spite of the fact that Jonathan was not even feeding very often, Becky had developed tender nipples. Giving up breastfeeding seemed to be the only solution. She was worried about her baby's weight, felt frustrated at every feed, and was exhausted from getting up every two hours to wake and feed him. One pediatrician watched her feed and checked her positioning, but noticed that although Jonathan appeared to go on the breast well, he gave a few weak sucks and stopped. The pediatrician could think of no reason for the baby's seeming disinterest, and brought Jonathan to see us.

We saw Becky nine days after birth. Her pediatrician came with her to see what she could learn, so she could help other women with Becky's problem. We first watched

Becky try to begin a feed. There were two problems with the way she was feeding Jonathan. One was that she was concentrating so hard on his positioning that she didn't think of her own. She chose to sit in a high-backed rocking chair, which was similar to the one she used at home. In this chair she leaned backward, and that pulled her breasts away from her baby. The other difficulty was that, although the position of the baby's mouth on her breast looked fairly good, his body was not tucked close enough into hers. The combination of these two problems, neither of them seemingly serious, had resulted in Jonathan not being able to take quite enough of her breast into his mouth, no matter how hard he tried.

Once Becky sat upright, with enough pillows to support her back and her baby's body as he lay on her lap, and once she held Jonathan tucked close into her, the change in his behavior was immediate! Instead of taking a few weak sucks and falling asleep or crying with frustration, he started to feed strongly and well. "It doesn't hurt at all!" Becky said, surprised. Jonathan fed for twenty-five minutes on one side and then let go of the breast. She sat him up for a minute to burp, and then she positioned him on her other breast. She wanted to learn to breastfeed lying on her side so we showed her how to do this. He took the second side just as well and let go when done. He fell asleep, full and contented.

Becky felt for the first time the joy of a problem-free, pain-free feed. After help to have one good feed, and an understanding of what had caused her problems, she went on to breastfeed her son well and with enjoyment. A week later Jonathan had gained half a pound in weight and this improvement continued.

Becky had difficulty in positioning Jonathan at her breast partly because she did not have good help in the early days after birth, but also because Jonathan was a sleepy baby, possibly because of the medication used during the birth. It is often the case that with sleepy babies the positioning has to be absolutely right, a small difference can prevent them from feeding.

If the breast is not in just the right place in the baby's mouth, the baby may not get the signals he needs. If he is put to the breast regularly, but is unable to feed well, he soon gets frustrated and cries, and then falls asleep while feeding, with the breast still in his mouth. This can become an impossible situation for both mother and baby. If not solved quickly, it can lead to a decision to bottle feed. It is easy to understand why.

Meili's Story:

Sore Nipples, Early Supplementing, and Return to Work with a Very Young Baby

*M*EILI was a mother of a six-year-old, expecting her next baby. She had had problems feeding Lily, her first. Lily had been eight weeks' premature, had been delivered by cesarean, and had spent six weeks in the special care nursery. Meili had used a breast pump at first to get her milk supply going, and Lily had been given her mother's milk; but when Meili had started to breastfeed Lily, she had developed sore nipples that had quickly become badly damaged and bled. She had stopped breastfeeding and gone back to using the breast pump, feeding Lily her breast milk from the bottle. After a week or two, she had stopped pumping too. "My milk just went," she told us. "I couldn't get any out."

In preparation for their second baby, Meili and her husband, Chin, went to childbirth classes. They wanted to have a normal birth this time. They also read a lot about breastfeeding. They arranged to use the money Meili had saved from her job to hire a full-time housekeeper for the first two weeks. Chin planned time off from work to be at home for the first ten days, so that together they could get the feeding right.

Meili went into labor at term with this child, but after nine hours the baby was found to be in a breech position. Meili was put on an intravenous drip in labor, and not allowed to drink anything. Meili was given a cesarean section with a spinal anesthetic (cesarean sections are often done today simply because the baby is breech, despite the fact that breech babies can often be safely delivered vaginally). After the cesarean she was given only ice chips to suck for the first two days. Meili was dehydrated and felt unwell for the first two days after the birth; she had a temperature and a sore throat. In spite of this difficult and disappointing beginning, Meili put her new baby, Peiwin, to her breast soon after birth and breastfed her. She fed lying down, as this was the most comfortable position for her after surgery.

From the second day on, Meili had sore nipples. Her husband, who had been told that to stimulate the milk supply a woman needs to breastfeed for at least fifteen minutes on each side, prompted her to keep feeding even though it hurt, and he timed each feed. Meili's nipples quickly became damaged and bled. By day four she had stopped breastfeeding, and had gone back to the pumping and bottle feeding she had used with her first child. When we saw them at home nine days after birth, both Meili and Chin expressed great disappointment that breastfeeding didn't work.

Meili's cesarean scar was healing well and her nipples were nearly healed. She was giving Peiwin bottles at every feed, alternating artificial milk with her breast milk, which she expressed by hand pump. She supplement with artificial milk, we learned, because Chin felt that perhaps she wasn't producing enough milk to feed the baby. The baby fed every two or three hours, and it was obvious that both parents were working hard to give her the best they could.

After we watched Meili put her baby on her breast, it was clear to us why she was having problems with her nipples. She sat in a comfortable chair to feed, but she was tense and bent forward over the baby, who lay on a pillow on her lap. Peiwin was not held close enough to her mother's body, and she lay more on her back than on her side. This meant she had to turn her head to find the breast. In addition, she didn't take enough breast in her mouth.

The baby was patient as Meili settled herself to feed. She went to the breast eagerly, but with her mouth not wide open enough, so her gums were fixed tightly over the nipple. Because Meili had large nipples and her baby had a small mouth (not an unusual combination for Asian mothers and babies), it was easy for Peiwin to take the nipple rather than the breast. Meili also was in the habit of keeping a finger on her breast, next to the areola, to keep the baby's nose clear. This tended to pull the breast back out of the baby's mouth. To compound the problems, Chin gave a constant stream of instructions as she fed.

Only small, but important, changes were need with what Meili was doing. First, she needed to sit more upright. Second, she needed to hold Peiwin's body facing hers and closer to her own. Third, she needed to brush Peiwin's lips with her nipple, wait for Peiwin's mouth to gape open wide, and then move the baby onto her breast.

Once she had these things described to her, Meili changed her position and tried to move Peiwin's open mouth onto her breast. She tried several times before getting it right. Then, for the first time, Peiwin drew Meili's nipple well back into her mouth and began to feed strongly and deeply. "It doesn't hurt at all!" Meili exclaimed, not quite believing it. As her baby continued to feed, she noted that although her nipple felt "funny"—as if it was being stretched—there was no pain. When her baby came off the breast, Meili noted with obvious delight that her nipple was not squashed flat, as it had been after all her other feeds, but was quite round.

"It was so nearly right, but not quite!" observed Chin, who had watched carefully. They both had explanations for why other helpers had not been able to fix the problem. Meili said, "The difference was that they did it for me! I was not even involved. They put her on and then left me to it. It helped to have your hand right over mind, guiding it—and then for you to watch me do it myself." Chin noted that the problem with breastfeeding books was that it was not possible to work out their particular problem from looking at a tiny diagram. "We needed a photograph of how it should be, along with a drawing, and a picture of what it looked like if it was wrong."

This was a classic case of how feeding could be almost right, but not quite, thereby ending up all wrong. A number of details were just a bit wrong: the mother's body position, the baby's body position, and the baby's mouth position on the breast. Together it added up to damaged nipples, a baby not getting the right balance of milk, and breasts not making enough milk, and a husband who had lost confidence in his wife's ability to breastfeed their baby. Added to this was the combination of a mother who was disappointed about having a possibly unnecessary repeat cesarean, a mother with large nipples, and a baby with a small mouth. The well-meaning but anxious concern of her husband made Meili nervous, and she had lost self-confidence.

We left their home after two hours, with Peiwin having had a good feed from both breasts (her first ever) and then having dropped off the breast after she was done, much to her mother's surprise. It had taken a few attempts by Meili to get her baby on right. We were careful to tell them both that it would take practice and a number of attempts before it would be quite right. There might well be one or two feeds where she wouldn't be able to get it right at all. But it would gradually get better as she and her baby learned. "Don't worry," we said. "You have the principles right. You just need practice, both of you."

We encouraged them not to have Meili pump her milk or supplement with artificial milk for the next few days. We told them to expect Peiwin to feed often, around the clock, for a few days, while she and her mother's milk supply caught up with each other. We encouraged them to call us if they needed help, but Meili and Chin assured us that hey would now manage by themselves.

A week later, when we checked by phone to see how Meili was doing, disappointment was in her voice as she said she was back to pumping and bottle feeding. She had had several good breastfeeds the day after we had seen her, but her nipples had become slightly sore as she had practiced getting her baby on right, and sometimes it hadn't worked. She had lost her confidence again, and even those good breastfeeds hadn't restored it. Chin had told her she should have toughened her nipples before the birth.

It seemed that Chin's concern, added to her lack of confidence (partly resulting from her feelings about her cesarean and partly from her first nine days of problematic feeding) made her unsure of her ability to breastfeed successfully. We offered again to come and sit with her for a feed and to observe and help her, or to find someone else who could come each day for a while, just to be a support while she practiced. She sounded delighted to hear that we were confident that she could get the baby back on the breast again, but she declined our offer to visit. Chin was still off work and it seemed he preferred to be her sole support. Because he was going to go back to work the next day, we suggested that Meili do her breastfeeding while she was alone, and supplement only while he was home, because his feeling that Peiwin was not getting enough milk led him to push Meili to supplement.

Meili agreed. She said she would like it if we would call her once in a while to see how she was doing. One of us called five days later and Meili said, "I've just lost all my confidence!" She had given up trying to breastfeed. The one day she had done it, the baby had gone on wrong once and within several strong sucks she had felt pain, so she hadn't tried again that feed. She had tried the next day, but Peiwin hadn't seemed interested in her breast, so she had given up.

Meili was still expressing milk, feeding Peiwin exclusively on her breast milk. But she had just been to see the pediatrician, who had told her that she was not giving her baby enough milk. "I just can't get more than 3 1/2 ounces from the pump," she said with great concern. We reminded her of how supplementing ended up decreasing her milk supply. We suggested that she continue to express milk often and try once again to breastfeed, but only when there was no one else in the house, because she did best when no one made her anxious. The baby, we said, would have to relearn to take the breast; it would just take time and patience, and care in getting her on right.

Meili did not continue to breastfeed, but she remained dedicated to her efforts to give Peiwin her milk. At one month Peiwin was growing well and was a contented baby. She fed from a bottle, having breast milk for all but one feed. Meili and Chin had worked out a creative solution between them that was satisfactory to Meili. She would express regularly during the day, beginning at 8:00 a.m. From the time Chin got home from work he would take over feeding Peiwin, and at the same time Meili would sit with them and express her milk for the next feed. She would express milk up until the 11:00 p.m. feed, and then after to get up only once more in the night to express milk. Chin got up with her at that time and fed Peiwin, and at 5:00 a.m., when Peiwin awoke for another feed, he would let Meili sleep and feed the baby a bottle of artificial milk. This arrangement worked for everyone, and it continued to work well for almost two more months, but then the demands upon Meili increased.

Meili had known that she would have to return to work only ten weeks after the birth because that was all the paid maternity leave granted by her company. There were no provisions for on-site day care, and employees were not permitted to work flexible hours to enable them to take time off during the middle of the day to go and breastfeed. Meili had planned to continue feeding Peiwin her breast milk; throughout the day she would use a breast pump to express milk and then refrigerate it. When it came time to make preparations to return to her job, however, Meili reassessed her choices and decided to wean Peiwin. Although her workplace is only a few miles from home, working meant she would leave the house at 8:00 a.m. and not return until after 5:30 p.m. Because of her position as accounting manager, Meili knew that she would have much work to catch up on and that she could not realistically plan to express milk while at work.

Meili wanted to make the transition as easy as possible for Peiwin and herself. She had carefully arranged that the day care person would be the same woman who had helped at the house part-time since Peiwin's birth. Meili decided that Peiwin would spend the day at the baby-sitter's house, which was nearby. This woman had two children of her own in high school and was very comfortable with young babies, especially Peiwin, whose needs she knew well by the time Meili returned to work. The baby-sitter had only one other child to care for, an eighteen-month-old boy, so Peiwin would have a great deal of cuddling and individual attention. To avoid painful engorgement from stopping breastfeeding suddenly, Meili weaned Peiwin onto formula over several weeks. The adjustment went well for both Peiwin and her mother, in part because Meili was comfortable with her child care arrangements and didn't feel guilty or anxious.

At her six-month checkup, Peiwin was pronounced strong, healthy, and big for a Chinese baby, which pleased her mother and father. She smiles easily and is good natured. She started sleeping through the night at six weeks, which made it much easier for Meili to return to work. To help Peiwin sleep, Meili and Chin tried to make sure that she had a large feed before bed-time. Each evening, after one of them bathed her, Peiwin would take a bottle of Meili's milk, but she would usually fall asleep after taking only a couple of ounces. Chin found that if he lay her down on her back, a position she usually didn't like, she would wake herself, and then he could feed her the rest of the bottle. (Note that parents are now encouraged to lay their babies on their backs to sleep, as this is the best position to prevent crib/cot death.) This strategy worked, and she continues to go to sleep without a lot of fussing, sometimes after talking to herself in her crib.

Meili combined traditional cultural advice and practices with modern assistance to make feeding work. She had worried that her breasts might not get enough stimulation from expressing milk to meet Peiwin's needs. She listed to her mother's advice and followed the ritual women in her ancestry had followed to assure an ample milk supply: "I made soup each day. Usually it was either a whole fish cooked in water with ginger and green onions, or pigs' knuckles cooked in water with peanuts. Otherwise I made chicken soup. I had these every day." Meili is not sure whether the soup made a differ-ence, but she felt comfortable following the traditional advice and is glad that she did. "I really tried very hard. It took a lot of work."

Meili wondered why breastfeeding had been so difficult for her. We suggested that it was not any one factor, but a number of things that added up to a considerable prob-lem. We reminded her how well she had done in the face of adversity, and she agreed; she is proud of her daughter and should take credit for how resourceful she and Chin have been. Meili gold us that if they have a third child she will definitely get help from the beginning to ensure she starts out right. "Then I think I will probably be able to breastfeed all the time," she said.

Judy's Story:
Too Much Milk

THREE years after giving up breast-feeding her baby in frustration, Judy was still feeling the disap-pointment. It is never possible to diagnose problems in retrospect, but Judy wanted to talk to us about what had happened to her, in order to gain some understanding of what had gone wrong. She hoped to have another baby, and very much wanted to breastfeed well. Judy had started leaking colostrum when she had been five month's pregnant, and had continued throughout her pregnancy. Her pregnancy had gone well and she had looked forward to birth.

She had had a normal labor, at term, and she had enjoyed giving birth. She told us proudly that she had pushed her daughter out in just thirty minutes. Clearly the birth had been a positive experience for Judy, unlike breastfeeding. The problems had begun when, after birth, the hospital staff had taken her baby, Jilly, to the nursery. Jilly had been hypoglycemic and without asking Judy's permission the staff had tried to insert an intravenous line into the baby to give her some glucose. When Jilly had been brought to Judy two hours later, her head was shaved and there were several punctures where someone had tried to insert the needle. "Why didn't they just let me feed her in the first place?" said Judy. "I had so much milk!" A nurse had helped her get breastfeeding started, and she had left the hospital without any idea that she would have any problems at home.

Jilly had then gone onto the breast and had fed well from the start. Judy had had no nipple problems, and Jilly had sucked strongly and effectively. She had awakened every two hours to feed, fed for fifteen to twenty minutes, and then gone to sleep. She had never wanted the second breast. She had grown quickly. By only three days after birth she had gained almost a pound, an unusual occurrence.

Judy's abundant milk supply had continued. One week after birth, Jilly had started to spit up some of every feed. A week later six of Judy's relatives, including her mother-in-law, had some to stay for two weeks. It had been Christmas, and Judy's in-laws had wanted to spend it with the new baby. This had caused problems for Judy and Dan, who had felt they had to look after their houseful of guests. Judy had become very tired, especially as Jilly still had been feeding every two hours.

At three weeks after birth, Judy had noticed her breasts were very full and heavy at each feed. She had started having to express milk before every feed, just so Jilly could take her breast. She remembered saying to her baby, "Please feed so my breasts won't hurt!" When she had been feeding,

she had leaked so much from the opposite breast that she had to hold a cup under the other breast or she would get soaked with milk.

Jilly had continued to bring up milk after each feed. At one month she had had two episodes of severe projectile vomiting. Because they did not happen again, and because Jilly had continued to gain one pound a week, Judy had continued to feed. By this time Jilly had often pulled off the breast and choked or gagged while feeding. It had looked to Jilly as if she was getting too much milk too fast. By this stage Judy had always been tired, unable to relax and enjoy feeds because of her full breasts, the leaking milk, and Jilly's choking and spitting up. She had turned to local breastfeeding counselors and health care workers for help, but no one had been able to tell her why she had so much milk.

All this time Jilly had been well and gaining weight fast—too fast for Judy's comfort. She had been a happy baby. Her stools had been quite normal, soft and yellow. Judy had gone back to work at ten weeks, and had expressed milk each day for her baby. Expression had been easy because she had had so much. The problem had been that it was hard to stay away from Jilly for any length of time, because Judy would quickly get full and sore.

Judy had breastfed for only three months, but, she said, "It felt like a year." Her life had been dominated by feeding and milk. With great regret she had put Jilly on a bottle and formula milk.

It is always hard to diagnose problems in retrospect, but there are several important clues in this story that point to Judy's simply having had too much breast milk. It had probably not been a problem of balancing the foremilk and hindmilk, because Jilly had always gone on well, finished the first breast first, and come off on her own. Also Jilly had had a normal stool, not the liquid, greenish stools that often indicate too much foremilk. It was not likely that it had been a positioning problem either. Judy had never had sore nipples or mastitis or any other indications of positioning difficulty. The baby had always taken her feeds in a reasonable length of time. Neither did it seem that it had been a letdown problem, because Judy had often found her breasts full, heavy, and leaking.

A very small number of women do produce too much breast milk. The first thing to do is to make sure that this really is the problem by ruling out the other causes. Often the problem resolves over two or three weeks. If not, then deliberately feeding from only one breast at each feed will limit breast stimulation and therefore milk supply. If all else fails, some women collect the excess milk and send it to the local breast milk bank.

Karen's Story:

Constant Feeding but a Slow-Gaining Baby, Mastitis, and a Diagnosis of Milk Intolerance

KAREN breastfed her first baby for ten months, in spite of having a range of problems, which included three episodes of mastitis. Her baby slept poorly at night and fed frequently, round the clock.

With Mark, her second baby, she hoped that breastfeeding would be easier, so that

she could enjoy her baby, rather than being constantly tired. She had a standard hospital birth, with a vaginal delivery but numerous routine interventions in labor. She started breastfeeding soon after birth, but found the first two feeds especially difficult, and received little help from the hospital staff. She developed sore nipples within the first week, but she did have occasional good, pain-free feeds. More often than not, however, she found feeding painful. "If only I had a good midwife to help me!" she said.

Karen's nipples healed enough that she was able to continue to breastfeed, but she rarely had a pain-free feed. Mark was not a contented baby. At thirteen weeks after birth, when we first saw them, he was almost a "failure-to-thrive" baby. He wanted to feed every hour, had green, liquid stools, and his weight gain was well below normal. Because of this he had a little, pinched face.

When we watched Karen feeding, it became clear that there was a positioning difficulty. She held Mark's body close to hers, and she waited for his mouth to open wide. But she bent over him, tense, with her shoulders hunched and chest curled inward, so that her breasts hung straight down toward her baby. Then, as she moved him onto her best, she bent the wrist of the hand supporting his head (Chloe calls the movement the flip), which bent his neck (it should be in a straight line with the back). This resulted in his chin dropping down toward his chest, a position that makes it almost impossible for a baby to feed well. It also buried Mark's nose in the breast, so Karen found she had to hold her breast out of the way so Mark could breathe.

Karen needed to learn to sit with her back erect (neither leaning back nor curled forward), and then to help Mark to take the breast straight on, rather than bending his neck inward as she put him on. She found it helped for her to support her breast, which slightly shaped it so that Mark could take the breast more easily (see page 46). She was able to relax into the feed because there was no pain at all. Mark fed well, with deep, long suckles, unlike the way he had been doing for the past three months. Mark came off the breast when he was done, looking sated, and Karen was greatly relieved.

With a new understanding of the basic principles of breastfeeding, Karen felt confident enough to go back home and continue on her own. She was delighted to discover that feeding did not hurt at all. Nor did she any longer need to hold her breast away from Mark's nose. We heard from her a week later that Mark's behavior had changed dramatically with that first good feed. He had slept soundly on the drive home and had fed well the rest of the day. He was sleeping well between each feed and beginning to feed less at night. He was gaining weight rapidly.

Karen had told us during her visit how she had learned about breastfeeding. She said that in her own career as a nurse, she had seen only problematic breastfeeding—never good, confident breastfeeding. She had seen bottle feeding, and she had a sense that what she had been doing was bottle feeding her baby with her breast. This meant that she had tried to put her breast into his mouth, rather than helping him to actively take her breast. She noted, "It's so easy to lose your confidence, even if you've done it wrong only once!"

She also talked about how problems with breastfeeding greatly affected the way women felt about breastfeeding. "So many of my friends want to breastfeed, but they've had problems with their first baby, and they just don't want to try it again." Karen believed it was important for women to have one-on-one skilled help when they need it, rather than just having the techniques shown to them and then being left on their own. She said it meant a lot to her that we had not done it for her, but had watched her body and her hands, had told her how to move them, and then had explained what had been right and what had been wrong with what she had tried.

We talked to Karen again when Mark was just over fifteen months old. She had continued breastfeeding him for nine months at which time he gradually weaned himself. Over a few weeks, he cut down from six feeds a day to just one at night, and then to one every two or three nights until he stopped completely.

When we asked about problems Karen had while breastfeeding, an interesting story emerged. She had had three episodes of mastitis, the first one starting when Mark was about five months old. "And I'm sure it wasn't a problem with positioning," she told us. "That problem was solved, but I still got mastitis." She was given antibiotics on two of the three occasions, but she also breastfed as often as she could. "I knew that the best treatment was to feed," she said. "It just felt like there was a blockage, and all we had to do was clear it."

The pattern of Mark's weight gain remained the same throughout the time he was breastfed, slow but steady. He was happy and healthy, and Karen received nothing but encouragement from the health workers. Her health visitor was especially supportive and kept in close contact. Karen was never advised by her health workers to supplement her breast milk with artificial milk or to stop breastfeeding, but Mark was watched carefully. Only two people suggested given Mark extra bottles. One was Karen's mother-in-law who had had an identical problem breastfeeding one of her children and who dealt with it by feeding from both the breast and the bottle. The other person was her husband who was worried about Mark's slow weight gain. Karen told us she suspected that he wanted a chance to feed the baby a bottle himself. When he did try, Mark refused it. "I would have given up breastfeeding if I had been advised to do that by my doctor or health visitor," she said. "But because they supported me, I did what I really wanted to do and kept feeding."

As soon as Karen started to introduce other foods, a new problem emerged. Mark simply refused to take milk products, so she gave him solids, juice, and water. She occasionally tried to give him formula milk after she stopped breastfeeding but did not force him to take it, and he consistently refused. She had the same result when she tried giving Mark ordinary cow's milk when he was a year old. At about fourteen months, Karen discovered that Mark would take a yogurt-based fruit drink. Soon after drinking it, however, he developed severe eczema, and an intolerance to cow's milk was diagnosed.

An intolerance to cow's milk explains the symptoms that Karen and Mark had experienced. The combination of a baby with slow weight gain in spite of efficient feeding and a mother with recurrent mastitis can indicate that the baby is intolerant to milk products. And a baby's refusal to take milk also points toward the baby's possible intolerance. In this case, a baby can be more perceptive than an adult.

As we talked with Karen, it became clear that both she and her husband have difficulty with milk products. Karen has eczema and her husband refuses all dairy products. Their older child, who had almost the same difficulties as Mark, is allergic to a number of foods, including eggs.

Karen told us her only real concern after the diagnosis was Mark's calcium intake. But recently he has started to drink soy-based milk with no ill effects; since it contains calcium, she is no longer worried.

"But I do wonder about breastfeeding another child if we have one," she said. Karen's doctor advised her not to breastfeed another baby, partly because she had found a lump in her breast, which felt somewhat like mastitis, two months after she stopped breastfeeding Mark. This gradually disappeared over about six weeks. Her doctor was concerned about the amount of mastitis she had experienced and suggested that she bottle feed if she has more children. Bottle feeding would be a problem, however, if the next baby was milk intolerant too, and there would be concern about what to feed him or her.

We suggested that with her next baby, she exclude all dairy products from her own diet. Since this is difficult to do, we told her to talk with her health visitor and a nutritionist. A baby can be intolerant of dairy products passed over in the breast milk, and the only way to solve this problem is to remove them entirely from the mother's diet.

Karen faced a difficult challenge breastfeeding her baby, and she dealt with it remarkably well. With good support from her health workers, she continued to breastfeed as long as her baby wanted. She did not force Mark to drink milk he did not want and, when the intolerance was diagnosed, made sure that he got a balanced diet. Although she was disappointed that breastfeeding was more difficult than she had imagined, she was aware that Mark would have had difficulty with milk substitutes. "I know it was the best thing to do, and I'm glad we succeeded," she said. "I just hope it's not so hard the next time."

Jenny's Story:

Getting It Right with the Third Baby, but Facing a New Challenge—Breastfeeding a Critically Ill Baby

*J*ENNY talked to us about her experience with Robbie, her nine-day-old son. She had been worried about breastfeeding, because she had had problems in the early days with Hugh and Tom, her first two children, who were now seven and three.

When she had had her first two babies, Jenny and her husband had been living in a part of the country where it was considered rude to breastfeed in public, or even to do it in front of guests in your own home. Jenny told us, "I always had to wait until visitors had gone or take the baby into another room." She had found this meant that she couldn't breastfeed when she and her baby needed to, and with each baby she had developed severe, painful engorgement a few days after birth. She also had had sore nipples for a few days.

The third time was different. They had moved across the country to a community

where breastfeeding was seen as a normal and natural way of feeding babies, and people were not shocked when a woman fed in public. Ever since the influx of young, progressive-minded people in the late 1960s, Santa Cruz—a college town on the coast in Northern California—has been a community where breastfeeding is an ordinary part of life.

Jenny started breastfeeding Robbie, who weight 8 pounds, 6 ounces at birth, shortly after he was born. She fed whenever he or she wanted to, whether she had visitors or was alone. She had no engorgement at all. She also said that she understood, without instruction, more about good positioning, as this was her third baby. Breastfeeding went smoothly and she never had sore nipples.

In Santa Cruz it is becoming common for women to spend the first month after birth at home, rather than moving right back into a busy life. This is a tradition in many cultures across the world, and helps to keep the world at bay. It honors a woman's need to have quiet time with her baby so she can recuperate and adjust to her new life. Jenny and Dave had decided during Jenny's pregnancy with Robbie to spend the first month of their new baby's life as quietly as possible. Jenny did not go out of the house at all for twenty-eight days, and Dave went out only to work and shop. Jenny said, "It's been wonderful: so relaxed and quiet."

Both Jenny and Dave commented to us that because their lives were usually so busy—with working, shopping, visiting, going out in the car, taking the older children out—it was hard to get the rest and time with a new baby that they and the baby needed. For Jenny and Dave, the way to deal with this was to cut down on anything that they did not have to do. They certainly looked relaxed and breastfeeding was going fine without any outside help.

Jenny had noticed that from birth Robbie breathed somewhat faster than had her other babies. She had pointed this out to the midwife and pediatrician and had been told that his breathing was within the normal range and, since his color was good and he was obviously thriving, there was no need for alarm. When Robbie was four months old, Jenny took him in for immunizations. At that time, the physician said he wanted to make sure Robbie's lungs were clear and suggested a chest x-ray. It was possible that Robbie had a minor form of bronchial asthma. The x-ray revealed the source of Robbie's rapid breathing: the lungs were clear, but the heart was quite enlarged. Jenny and Dave were told that Robbie would have to be admitted to the hospital for further tests to find the cause of the enlargement.

Robbie was admitted that evening, a happy, healthy looking baby, and Jenny and Dave remained at his side throughout the night. At first a virus was suspected, but when a recording of the heartbeat was done, the situation proved much more serious: the coronary artery was attached to the pulmonary side of the heart. Robbie was transferred by ambulance to the nearest hospital that performed heart transplants, and the next morning he went into surgery, smiling. The two older boys were sent to stay with a relative temporarily so Jenny and Dave could give all their attention to Robbie. His heart was operated on and he was taken off the bypass machine, but his heart would not begin beating. He

was put onto full life-support systems until that afternoon when, miraculously, a heart became available in Texas.

Robbie survived a complete heart transplant, the hospital's 528th and second youngest transplant patient to do so. Surgeons, cardiologists, and nurses told Jenny that it seemed likely that Robbie was thriving because he entered surgery in such good condition. They acknowledged that breastfeeding may have played an important part. Jenny resumed full breastfeeding three days after the transplant when the respirator was removed and Robbie breathed on his own. She continued to breastfeed throughout his three week stay in the hospital and learned that Robbie was the first child known to have been breastfed after a transplant. Because no research had been done on breastfeeding a baby who had had a heart transplant, the surgeon was concerned that Jenny's breast milk may contain certain immune factors that could cause Robbie's body to reject his new heart. This is the greatest danger faced after a heart transplant. A medical conference was held but no good reason cold be found for Jenny to stop breastfeeding, and she was permitted to continue. The physicians' second concern was how to monitor the amount of nourishment Robbie received by breast. It is extremely difficult to measure the amount of milk a breastfed baby receives, so they observed Robbie closely. All outward signs of his health supported Jenny's decision to breastfeed.

Jenny breastfed Robbie day and night, and he had no artificial feeding at the hospital. She carried a beeper that the nurses used to call her every time he was hungry. "My milk would let down each time the beeper went off!" Jenny said. This was inconvenient at times, especially when it went off by mistake, but Jenny was committed to breastfeeding. "I felt that it was the best thing for him. I'd nursed him from birth. I almost lost my milk the first days he was in the hospital because I couldn't nurse. But I kept pumping and telling myself I had to keep my supply up so that when Robbie was able to take my milk, it would be there."

Robbie recovered quite rapidly and without complication. Everyone at the hospital commented on the importance of the special contact that Jenny provided by breastfeeding Robbie in the hospital. Members of the hospital team had warned Jenny prior to surgery that if Robbie survived, his development would regress and he would be like a newborn. And just like a newborn, he benefited from the skin-to-skin contact with his mother.

Today Robbie is eight months old and back at home with his family. It has been four months since the heart transplant, and Robbie is healthy and active again, crawling and standing and beginning to talk. He continues to receive immunosuppresant drugs daily to prevent the rejection of his new heart. He now eats organically grown, commercial baby food but continues to breastfeed as often as he wants. Robbie's breastfeeding and his amazing recovery have been the topic of discussion at many medical conferences and at hospital rounds across the country. Jenny advises any mother whose breastfeeding baby must be hospitalized for any reason to 'continue breastfeeding, no matter what it takes. I went through some hard times, and I lost a lot of sleep. You might too, but it is well worth it."

Juanita's Story:
Twins

WE met Juanita when her twin boys, José and Pablo, were three and a half weeks old. We had asked a local breastfeeding consultant if there was a mother of twins we could visit. Juanita had said she'd be glad to let us photograph her feeding. We had not been told of any feeding problems before we saw her.

Juanita had had a cesarean section with an epidural anesthetic at term, because she had not been able to find an obstetrician who would deliver her twins vaginally (even though this remains a normal practice in many countries). The babies had been healthy and well nourished in the womb: José had been 6 pounds 13 ounces and Pablo had been 6 pounds. Juanita had come home from the hospital within a few days. She and her husband had immediately found someone to come and help at the house during the day for the first month, so she could just be with her babies, breastfeed, and try to rest.

She had lots of support from her local support group for parents of twins and from the mother-to-mother breastfeeding group in her area, The Nursing Mothers Council. In the hospital she had received little help from the staff. She felt this had been due to poor communication between the nurses and herself: "I had a constant battle with the nursery staff," she told us. "They would take the babies away and tell me I needed to rest. Then I would find out that the babies had been formula fed in the nursery because the staff had been too busy to bring them back to my room."

Juanita had recovered quickly from her cesarean, but had been quite tired from being up at all hours with José and Pablo. She had tried to sleep as much as she could between feeds. Her husband, Frank, had been very supportive of her breastfeeding and had praised her for her mothering of the boys.

By the time we met Juanita and her babies, José was doing well but Pablo had gained little weight since birth. He was bright and woke regularly for feeds, but Juanita had problems putting him on her breast, and he was often fussy and seemed disinterested in feeding after a short time on the breast. Because he was fussy and José was not, Juanita found herself blaming Pablo at times for his behavior, even though she knew it was not really his fault. When tired and worried because breastfeeding isn't going right, a mother can often blame herself or her baby, not realizing that the problem has to do with the feeding itself.

Both babies had had an episode of thrush at two weeks (probably caused by the antibiotics that Juanita had been given as a matter of routine before her cesarean to prevent postpartum infection from the surgery). The doctor had planned to treat only the babies for thrush, but Juanita had understood that it would be a problem if she got thrush on her nipples, so she had asked for treatment for her nipples too. The thrush had cleared in a week.

Juanita knew about breastfeeding because her mother had breastfed all of her thirteen children. She had the confidence to withstand comments that she got from other people. "I keep getting told not to let them feed longer than twenty minutes," she said. Mothers are often given advice, especially mothers of twins! Juanita had also been told

by several people always to feed both babies at the same time so that it would take less time. But she had decided that until breastfeeding was established and both babies were feeding well, she wanted to feed them separately and concentrate on one baby at a time.

First we watched José, the bigger baby, feed. He did well, but we were able to show Juanita how to change the positioning of José's mouth on her breast so he could feed well in less time.

Pablo was the smaller baby, and it was clear that he was one of those small, sleepy babies who needed to have everything in the right place to give him exactly the right stimulus to feed. Several details needed close attention. First, a pillow down behind her back helped Juanita to straighten her posture. This brought her breasts forward and tilted her nipples slightly down, rather than flattening them and tilting the nipples up, the way they had been when she had leaned back. Changing the position of her arms also helped.

She started to feed with Pablo's head in the crook of her arm, but this seemed to give her little control over his head and neck. This is especially important with small babies. We suggested switching arms, putting her baby in the arm opposite from the breast. This way her hand was across his shoulders, cradling his head, allowing Pablo to be well supported along his upper back, neck, and head. Juanita said that she found it easier to help him get well positioned this way. Pablo then needed to be moved quickly onto the breast when he opened his mouth wide.

Juanita also needed to pay special attention to Pablo's lower jaw. It needed to be planted firmly on the underside of her breast as he opened his mouth, so that he took enough of the breast into his mouth.

She did this and Pablo got a good mouthful of breast and started to feed deeply, strongly, and well. He gulped the milk and was finished quite soon, letting his mother know this by coming off the breast. He went onto the other breast after a few tries, and fed deeply and quickly from it too.

While Pablo was learning to go to the breast well, José began to cry loudly, in spite of the fact that he had come off the breast contented not long before. Despite being cuddled he continued crying until his twin brother started to feed well; then José instantly calmed himself.

In the next weeks Juanita found that she still needed practice to get it right, especially with Pablo, but it gradually got better. It got to the point where she was confident enough to feed both babies at the same time when necessary, and Pablo was steadily gaining weight and filling out.

We spoke to Juanita when the twins were seven and a half months old, and both she and the boys were thriving. The boys were good natured and weighed almost 18 pounds each. The pronounced differences in size and development that were so striking when we first saw them, when Pablo was having difficulty at the breast, were gone. Juanita was still breastfeeding, usually feeding both at the same time, which made life simpler for everyone. For the first four months the boys had seldom slept or fed at the same time, meaning Juanita could not count on more than two or three hours of unbroken sleep!

"It's definitely been worth it to breastfeed this long, and I'll continue for as long as we all are enjoying it. It has been diffi-

cult," Juanita said, "but what helped me was using a breast pump whenever I needed to leave the boys for an afternoon or when I needed to get four or five hours of unbroken sleep. I rented an electric pump and used the attachment that allowed me to pump both sides at the same time. At times when I did pump I would have to use it every hour or two to keep my supply up. But it worked."

Juanita and the boys did not establish a regular feeding schedule until the twins were seven months old. At four months Juanita had tried giving cereal once a day, hoping it might help them sleep through the night. "The books I'd read said that wouldn't do it; and they were right, it didn't." But the boys, José in particular, enjoyed having a little cereal each morning after feeding, so Juanita continued. At six months José and Pablo started refusing bottles of pumped milk; Juanita felt this was because they liked breastfeeding so much more. They did, however, enjoy drinking a little juice or water from a cup. At seven months they began sleeping through most nights.

Juanita now breastfeeds around 6:30 a.m. and again at 10:00 a.m. The boys also eat a little cereal at one of the morning feeds. They get snacks of fruit or other solid food after their lunch feed and then breastfeed again around 2:30 p.m. If she wants to go out for the afternoon, she leaves them with a baby-sitter who gives them juice or yogurt. Juanita breastfeeds once more in the late afternoon and at that time gives them cereal and a vegetable. Just before bedtime Juanita breastfeeds them once more.

A few weeks ago Juanita thought she might have a breast infection; it was the first problem she had had breastfeeding.

One nipple was very sore during feeding. When it didn't clear up after a few days, she went to a clinic and the cause was discovered—a pimple on the nipple. It was recommended that she stop nursing and pump that side until the pimple cleared, but Juanita didn't feel comfortable with the advice. "Once I found out it was not a breast infection and realized that even if the pimple burst the pus would not cause the boys any problems I wasn't concerned." Successful breastfeeding seems to have played a large part in her self-confidence; she knows when to see advice but feels fully capable of evaluating whatever advice she gets.

Kathy's Story:

Inverted Nipple, Large Breasts

KATHY'S baby, Sarah, was three months old when we met the family. We had arranged to see them to talk about Kathy's experience of breastfeeding with an inverted nipple. What we saw was a wonderful example of creativity with breastfeeding when faced with serious difficulty.

Kathy had already breastfed her son, Ben, now eleven years old. After a home birth with no complications, she had started breastfeeding. This had been challenging; her right nipple had been fine, just a bit flat at the beginning. But her left nipple had been turned completely inward. It had not improved at all during pregnancy, when many flat and inverted nipples protrude

more because of the hormones of pregnancy.

When she had started breastfeeding, Kathy had tried to feed on the side with the inverted nipple, and found that her baby simply could not manage to take her breast. But Kathy had not been worried. Her mother had been with her to help, and she had had the same problem—with all of her seven healthy breastfed children! She had fed all of them, including twins, on one side only. As the eldest of the family, Kathy had seen this and considered it to be quite normal.

So she had breastfed Ben on one side only, with no supplements, until five months. She had finally stopped breastfeeding altogether at ten months. "I missed it when he stopped," she told us.

Sarah's birth, also at home, had been just as straightforward. Kathy had tried again to breastfeed on the side with the inverted nipple, but had found that it was still not possible. So she had fed on her right side only. She had found that the side she was not using became very engorged (swollen up under her arm), tender, and hot to the touch on the third day after birth, "But I expected it and I knew it would get better. It cleared up by the next day." The side she had been feeding from had not become engorged.

For the first week she had had a sore nipple on the side from which she fed. This, she had realized, was because she had to relearn positioning. "I also had a very sore back," she remembered, "and I would slump over Sarah as I was feeding her. The sore nipple got better when my back improved and I could sit up in a straighter position."

Kathy's other challenge was that she had large, soft breasts. But she had discovered that all she had to do was support her breast underneath with one hand throughout the feed. "The only problem is that I can't feed her and do something else at the same time," she told us, "because I need to use both hands. But that means I get to sit down and rest."

At three months after birth, when we talked, Kathy and Sarah were relaxed and happy with breastfeeding. Sarah would feed for as long as she wanted, and then come off to burp and play for a few minutes. Then she would go back on the same side again for another feed, until she came off herself. "I never tried to time her feeds," Kathy recalled. "My mother never did!"

Kathy had plenty of milk on one side. Sarah fed enthusiastically and well, and came off content. Her weight gain was good, and she was bright and alert. "I am a bit lop-sided," Kathy said with a smile. "It took a couple of months for the breast I am not using to stop leaking a lot of milk. Now it leaks just a little and it is much smaller than the side I do use. But that's not a problem!" Kathy knew that when she stopped breast-feeding, both breasts would end up much the same size (although no woman's two breasts are precisely the same size or shape).

Kathy talked to us about the feelings she had had about her inverted nipple as a teenager. "I thought I was deformed," she said. Although she smiled, it obviously had been a serious concern for her as a very young woman.

She also told us the story of her sister, Frances, who had recently had her first child. Frances had wanted to breastfeed, but she had very inverted nipples on both sides. In spite of skilled and constant care from Kathy, her mother, and her midwife, Frances had not been able to get her baby to take the breast on either side. "She tried so hard her nipples were sore and bleeding," Kathy told us. "But after three weeks she realized it would not be possible, and decided to pump her breast milk and feed it by bottle." This was a solution that worked for Kathy's sister, even though it was not ideal.

Although many women can breastfeed with inverted nipples, there are some who simply cannot get the baby to take the breast. Kathy's story of feeding on one side, her mother's story of feeding twins on one side, and her sister's story of pumping and feeding expressed milk were all thoughtful, creative examples of how to overcome serious difficulties.

"I'm so pleased that I've been able to breastfeed," Kathy told us as we left. "It's no trouble when we go out: no bottles of milk. She just feeds quietly under my blouse or a shawl wherever we are. She's a take-along baby!"

Sarah was nine months old when we last spoke to Kathy. Breastfeeding was continuing to go smoothly and there had been no problems. At five and a half months Kathy noticed Sarah was fussy after almost every feed, so she began giving her solid foods at that time. Sarah now takes the breast only once or twice in the morning and once before bed. She's been sleeping through most nights for the past month, but on nights when she does awaken, Kathy breastfeeds her. She plans to continue breastfeeding until Sarah is about a year old.

"The times I breastfeed her are so nice and relaxing for both of us. I think I'd miss it if we stopped now. It's the only thing that only I can do for her!"

Nada's Story:
Several Episodes of Mastitis

WHEN Robin, my second baby, was 3 weeks old I'd already had mastitis twice. Since I had fed my first baby, Lily, without any major problems, this came as a great shock. Admittedly, I did have sore nipples for the first couple of weeks with my first baby but I thought that was normal. Lily didn't choose to stop feeding until 16 months in a very easy and natural way.

When I became pregnant with Robin the last thing I had any concern about was breastfeeding, because I knew I could do it. I was much more concerned about Lily's reaction to the new baby because she was now a very active two and a half year old and I didn't want her to feel pushed aside.

When Robin was born I was surprised by his tiny little body, though he actually weighed eight and a half pounds! I expected him to behave as Lily had done during those many happy months of trouble-free feeding. But he didn't. I had to ask for help for the first few feeds. I was reminded how to entice him to open his mouth wide to take in the breast, and how to hold him so that he was opposite my breast and not in the crook of my arm.

I took him home when he was just over a day old. Lily was delighted. She wanted to hold him and kiss him. I was very relieved. I was very pleased that I did not have sore nipples this time and, looking back, I think I became a bit careless about positioning. I probably was concentrating more on Lily when I was feeding because I wanted her to be happy.

I started my first bout of mastitis on the seventh day. First I felt shivery and my right breast felt a bit tender. I didn't understand what was happening and continued to feed normally. By the afternoon I noticed that my breast had a reddened area where it had been tender and I had a definite fever. I knew this meant that I had mastitis. Everything that I had read about breastfeeding said that I must see a doctor. Luckily, my husband was still at home and we managed to arrange a visit to our family doctor. He prescribed antibiotics but also told me to continue feeding on the affected side. By the time I went to bed I felt much better. The redness had started to disappear and my temperature was going down. I assumed that I had an infection and that would be the end of the problem.

In the middle of Robin's third week I was dismayed to find that my right breast was beginning to be uncomfortable again. I didn't want to have more antibiotics but I didn't know what else to do to stop mastitis from developing . So far I wasn't feeling as ill as last time, so I quickly arranged to visit my doctor. Now that I was on my own at home with the children I did not want to feel as ill again. It was awkward because I had to take both children with me. My doctor again prescribed antibiotics and this time it seemed to stop any further progression of the mastitis.

I was puzzled by the fact that the problem had only occurred in my right breast but I knew that Robin was always a bit more fussy on that side as well. Two more weeks passed before I became suspicious that the right breast was beginning to feel as though I was going to get yet another bout of mastitis. This time I definitely did not want to take more antibiotics. I had luckily met another mother who had had similar problems and she told me about a breastfeeding clinic.

I was pleased to be told that they could see me that day. The only stipulation was that I should arrive when I thought Robin was going to be ready to feed so that we could be observed. I was also told that I could, if necessary, take Lily too, as the clinic had plenty of toys. Luckily, a friend of mine had invited her to play with her children.

When I got to the clinic a brief history of my problem was taken. I was told the mastitis might be due to the way the baby was attaching to that breast. The breastfeeding specialist wanted to observe this. Robin woke about twenty minutes after I arrived and I was taken into the clinic room. I was asked to begin by feeding on the right side. Once she had watched Robin go on she said she was pretty sure that she knew why there was a problem. She pointed out that Robin's bottom lip was too close to the base of my nipple which meant that his tongue could not draw the breast deeply enough into his mouth. This meant that he would not be able to remove the milk effectively from all parts of my breast. I was asked to remove him gently from the breast and try again. But this time I was to concentrate on placing his bottom lip as far away from the base of the nipple as I could, and to get his lip and chin to the breast first. She explained that it was his tongue and jaw which did all the work. I did what she said and I could tell immediately that he was feeding more effectively, because I could feel the difference.

As the feed continued I received further explanation. When Robin wasn't well

attached to the breast, milk would have been retained in the part of the breast that he had not emptied well. Some of the milk components would have leaked into the surrounding tissue. This would have set up an inflammatory response, which is what most mastitis is. Antibiotics probably have an anti-inflammatory effect, so the breast would improve, but antibiotics clearly hadn't stopped it from happening again. She said that research has also shown that mastitis most commonly occurs on the side opposite the mother's preferred holding side. This was right for me, because I always carry and cuddle my babies on the left. I remembered that it was always my right nipple that had been more sore when Lily was a baby.

At last I had an explanation and a plan to help prevent a recurrence. For the next few days I paid great attention to attaching Robin to my right breast correctly, in spite of the distractions from Lily. It became easier each day and soon I was able to stop thinking about it.

Robin is now six months old and I have had no further mastitis. I feel pretty confident that it will not happen again. It was a great relief to learn that there was an explanation and especially that I could do something to prevent it happening again.

Simone's Story:
Possible "Breast Rejection"

I was taught how to put my baby Geoffrey to the breast while I was in hospital, and I felt quite confident. But I never found breastfeeding truly relaxing and peaceful because Geoffrey was never calm while feeding. He grew well, which felt very satisfying, and he slept quite well at night. But he wriggled and pulled away a lot during feeds.

But his daytime feeds became more and more difficult. By the time he was three months old, he would feed for a few seconds, then pull away from the breast screaming and writhing in discomfort. Sometimes my milk seemed to gush out so fast that he would come away coughing and spluttering, milk spraying everywhere. It was very upsetting for both of us. Feeding him in public became impossible because of my embarrassment.

I had heard that there was a breastfeeding specialist in our local maternity hospital. I was told she was happy to see older babies too. I had become so concerned that I arranged to take Geoffrey to see her. I was afraid that he might become so distressed that he might refuse to go to the breast at all.

I timed my drive to the hospital so that he would be ready to feed when I got there. The specialist said she wanted to see how he went to the breast. When he woke I put him on. She noticed immediately that he was so far across my body that his head was tipped forwards making his tongue and jaw too far away from the breast. She suggested that I slid him slightly away from the breast he was feeding from and towards the middle of my body. This resulted in his head straightening up and his jaw and tongue coming much closer to the breast. Within a few minutes Geoffrey was feeding quietly and calmly! When he had finished, he came away from the breast, sat up, burped and actually smiled. Because I found it difficult to believe that such a small change could have affected his behavior in such a dra-matic way, I asked if I could return in a day or two just to make sure I was getting it right.

From that very feed, Geoffrey's behavior improved dramatically. When I went back for a second visit the midwife complimented me on how well I was doing. He has been such a happy boy since then. I can now feed him wherever I want and I now look forward to feeding him instead of dreading it.

Lin's Story:
Early Breast Refusal or "Fighting at the Breast"

MY baby Sharon was born by cesarean section after I had been in labor for a long time. Luckily I already had an epidural anesthetic in place, so I was awake when she was born. But I was unable to hold her myself for quite some time afterwards because of the intravenous drip in my right arm and my fear that I might fall asleep and drop her.

I had always known that I would breastfeed my baby and was looking forward to the first feed. I was sad that my hospital required that the first feed should take place within two hours of birth. If it didn't Sharon would be given formula. Around two hours after she was born, someone came to help me feed Sharon, though she hadn't yet shown any sign of hunger.

I found it a very distressing experience. I was helped to turn partly onto my side. Sharon's head was held firmly and she was pushed onto my breast. She cried but made no effort to open her mouth wide. The more times she was pushed, the more she cried. This was not at all how I had imagined our first feed would be. When it became obvious that she wasn't going to feed she was put back into the cot while the formula was fetched and given by bottle.

About three hours later I saw Sharon starting to turn her head from side to side and opening her mouth. I called for help and unfortunately the same nurse came back. Again, her head was held firmly and she was forced onto my breast. This time it seemed as though she was trying to pull away as well as crying throughout the attempt. I began to feel as though she was rejecting me and this, added to the discomfort I was now feeling from my wound, was very distressing. Unfortunately my husband was not there to comfort me because he had gone home to have a well-earned sleep.

Sharon and I were lucky that a more skilled person was called to see if she could help. She held Sharon gently, talking to her and calming before trying again. She let Sharon's lips brush my nipple and waited for her to open her mouth. Whenever she started to cry, the nurse would hold her and calm her before trying again. On the third attempt she succeeded and Sharon started to feed steadily and calmly. She stayed at my breast for about half an hour and came off all by herself. She looked so relaxed we decided to leave her alone for a while and not offer the other breast. I felt tired but very much happier.

When Sharon next looked hungry I decided to see if I could help her by myself. My intravenous drip had been taken out so I asked if I could be helped to sit up. It was difficult to sit up straight because my wound was so sore but I decided to try anyway. I was pleased that she seemed much calmer

than at the beginning of he two previous feeds. She opened her mouth several times but I was unable to latch her on by myself. Another nurse came to help and Sharon attached to my breast this time without even crying at all.

I needed some help for most feeds over the next two or three days but was delighted to find that it became easier all the time, even though it was quite a challenge when my breasts filled up. I don't like to remember those distressing early feeds but am so happy that she is now a thriving and contented baby.

Shenaz's Story:
"Colic"

ALI is my first baby. We had been married nine years before we decided to try for a baby and three years later (I was now 35) we got worried and arranged to visit a fertility clinic. As sometimes happens, by the time my appointment arrived, I had just missed a period.

My pregnancy was normal and I was thrilled to have a normal delivery in spite of my age. I had wanted this baby so badly. Feeding got off to a pretty good start, though, my nipples were very sore during the first week.

Things began to get more difficult as the weeks went by. Ali's feeds had always been very long and he would fall asleep at the breast. He fed very often, both day and night. He passed a lot of wind and his stools were wet and bubbly. Sometimes he fed noisily as if he was swallowing air, but he seemed to find it difficult to burp. But the worst thing was his crying. It happened after most feeds but got worse as the day went on. When I asked for help, I was told that I didn't have a problem because he was growing so fast. Admittedly he was averaging 8 to 10 ounces a week, and I knew that I had more than enough milk.

I was doing everything I could for Ali but he was so unhappy. He certainly wasn't the dream baby I had hoped for. I started asking family and friends for advice. My grandmother told me I was overfeeding him, but I couldn't work out how I could do anything about that. My best friend said it could be something I was eating and suggested I cut out cows' milk. I tried that for a week, but it didn't make any difference at all. Ali was now 6 weeks old and I was beginning to get desperate.

Luckily another friend suggested that I see a lactation consultant whom she knew had helped a mother with a colicky baby. I made an appointment and hoped that Ali would demonstrate his distressing behavior while I was there. I hadn't realized that the consultant would need to see him feed. I finally managed to wake him by changing his diaper and put him to the breast. She observed that I was trying to center the nipple halfway between his lips as if I was bottle feeding and I was also trying to put my breast into his mouth.

With simple suggestions and information she helped me change the way I was positioning him so that he could draw my breast more deeply into his mouth. The sucking felt more gentle and he paused more often. The feed was much quieter that usual. But the biggest surprise was that he let go all by himself after about 10 minutes—and looked contentedly asleep. I held him up for a moment and he did a neat little burp and remained quiet and relaxed. I was sure that he could not have had enough in such a short time but the consultant explained why there had been such a dramatic change. I was urged to return if there was not a steady improvement. I should expect my milk supply to settle down and his stools to become less liquid and less frequent. But we had no more problems. This was my dream baby.

For the first time I had an explanation that not only made sense but had obviously changed Ali's behavior.

Here is what she told me:

"The first milk in a feed is high in volume and low in fat. If the baby is helped to remove the milk more effectively it gets creamier as the feed proceeds. In this way the baby gets more calories in less time and comes away sooner when satisfied. The right mixture of milk affects what happens in his large bowel. A large feed of milk that doesn't contain enough cream causes gas to form (and the stools to be loose) and this causes pain. Because he needed a lot of milk to grow, the breasts replace the large feeds a baby takes by continuing to make lots of milk."

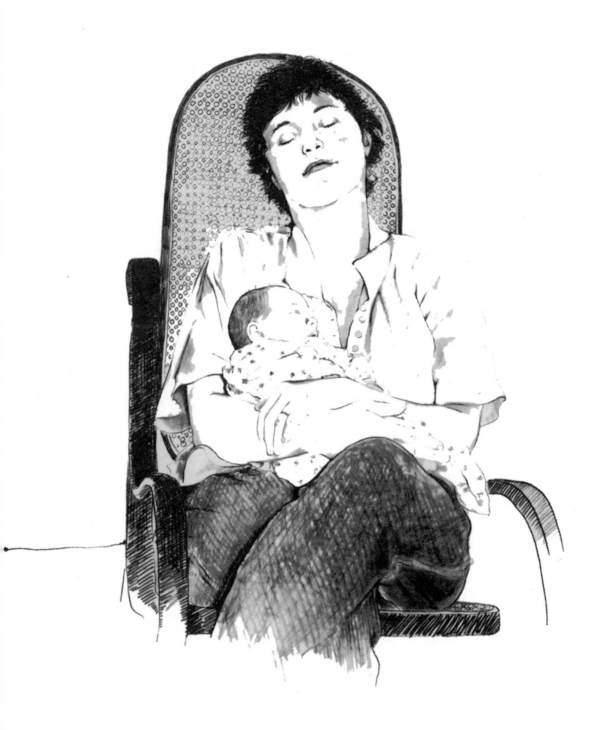

CHAPTER NINE

The Ten Basic Steps: A Storyboard

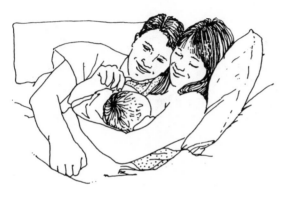

Step 1:

Breastfeeding is best for women, babies, and families.

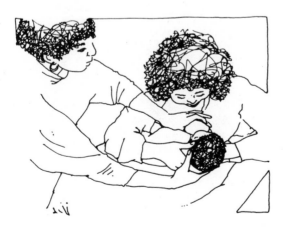

Step 2:

It is important to find good, skilled help for the first weeks after the baby is born—to help you get breastfeeding started well, and to help around the house.

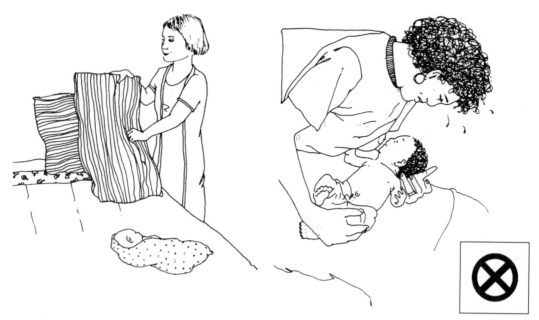

Step 3:

Before you begin, think about your posture and your baby's posture.

First, you need to get yourself comfortable. Breastfeeding is something that is learned, and like anything you learn it may take time and practice for both you and your baby to do it well.

Don't let yourself be in an uncomfortable position when you breastfeed. That will make you tense or tired.

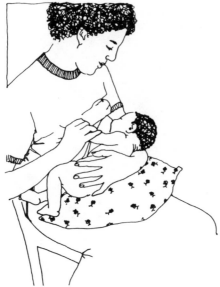

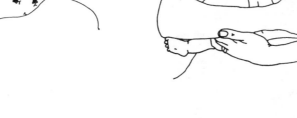

Next, make sure your body is in a good position for feeding—back straight (upright if you are sitting) and your breast free.

Hold your baby very close so the entire front of her body—and her head—are facing you, tucked up next to your body.

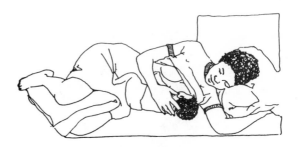

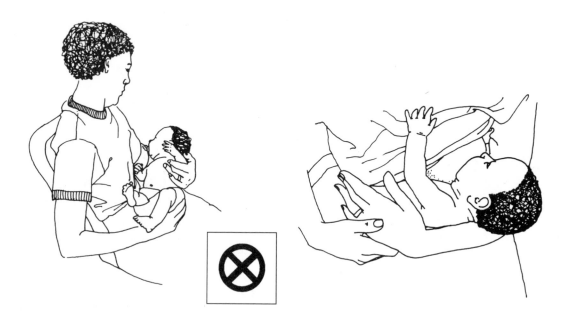

Don't make her have to turn her head to take the breast; it is very difficult for her to feed that way.

Put your baby so that her nose is level with your nipple when her mouth is closed. That way when she takes your breast her lower jaw will be pressed against your breast. If you hold her in your arms, let her head lie on your forearm.

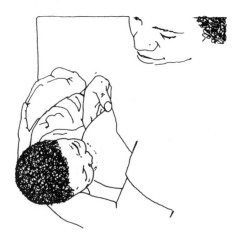

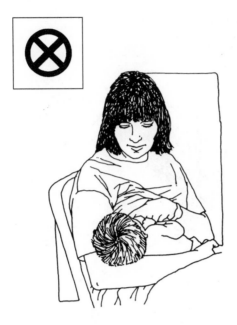

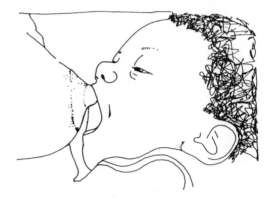

Don't hold her too far to the side or any way that pulls on your breast. Don't have her head in the crook of your arm or she will be to the side of your breast as she feeds.

Wait until she gapes her mouth wide open before bringing her on to your breast.

Bring the baby to the breast, not the breast go to the baby. Don't try to place your breast into her mouth, as if your breast were a bottle; instead put her onto your breast.

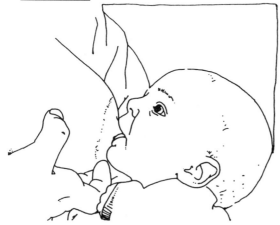 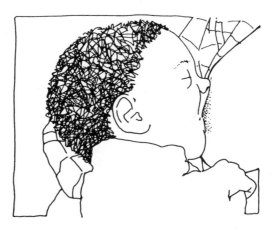

Don't let her just take her nipple in her mouth. It is breast feeding, *not* nipple feeding.

If your baby does not take enough breast into her mouth, then gently break the suction, using your finger to release your nipple, and take her off and try again.

Make sure she takes a large enough mouthful of breast, not only the nipple. If she takes enough breast into her mouth then your nipple will not get sore.

Be patient with yourself and with your baby. Take whatever time you both need!

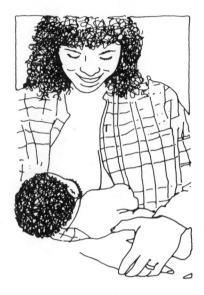

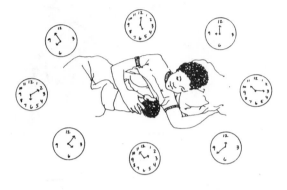

Step 4:

Breastfeeding should not hurt you! For a while, there may be a quick stab of pain as your baby begins to feed. But if pain continues for more than a few seconds, gently take her off and try again.

Step 5:

Your baby will need to feed often (more often than a baby on artificial milk) throughout the day and also during the night, in the first few weeks. She will not feed at any regular time for a while, but eventually she will settle into a regular schedule.

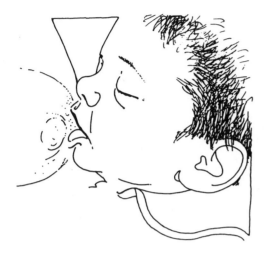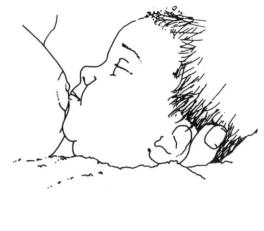

Step 6:

She will suck deeply and regularly most of the feed and come off the breast by herself when she is finished. Let her show you when she has had enough. Note: Your baby may stop suckling a few times during a feed and then start again. That is normal.

Let your baby come off the breast herself when she has had enough. Don't take her off the breast just because you think the clock tells you she should be done.

Remember occasionally to give her the chance to burp/wind after each feed.

If you or your baby becomes frustrated or upset, stop. Calm yourself. Calm your baby. Then try again.

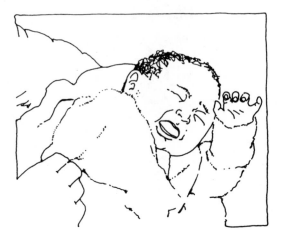

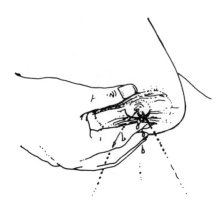

Step 7:

If your baby cries a lot at the breast—or often cries for a long time after a feeding—or if she does not continue to gain weight, she may not be feeding well. To be sure, first go back over Concepts 2, 3, 4, and 5 and see if you can improve positioning.

If you have a difficult time getting the baby to feed well on your breast, ask someone to look at these pictures and watch you while you put the baby on your breast to see if you are doing everything correctly. Sometimes it is hard to see for yourself, and a helper can be important.

Step 8:

Learn how to hand express your milk or how to use a breast pump for times when you cannot breastfeed, so that your baby can always have your milk.

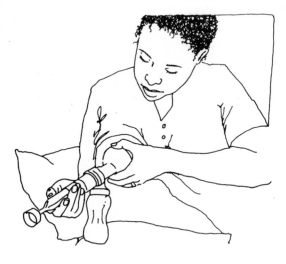

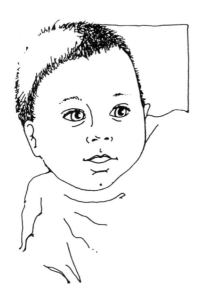

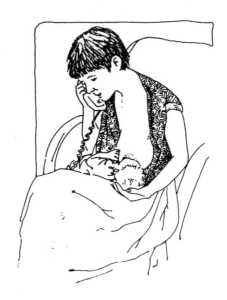

Step 9:

You will know your baby is thriving if she is gaining weight and looking healthy. If your baby is doing well, she will need no bottles of artificial formula or extra food until at least six months.

Step 10:

If you become sick, or if you feel your baby may be sick, *continue giving her your breast milk* and contact a health worker immediately.

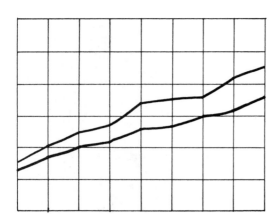

A Final Word

WE hope this book, with its suggestions and stories of breastfeeding women, will help you to breastfeed your baby well and happily. If this book has been helpful, please share it with someone else who might need it. The three of us have learned most of what we know from women like you who have breast-fed, and we are confident that women can teach each other about getting breast-feeding right, once they have good information.

The ability to breastfeed is a special and powerful attribute. Breastfeeding well will result in women having increased confidence in themselves and their bodies. We look forward to the future generations of happily breastfed babies and confi-dent breastfeeding women.

About the Authors, Photographer, and Illustrator

Mary Renfrew

Mary Renfrew is Professor of Midwifery Studies at the University of Leeds, England and is Director of the Mother and Infant Research Unit there. She was born in 1955 and educated in Scotland, graduating from the University of Edinburgh with a degree in nursing and social science.

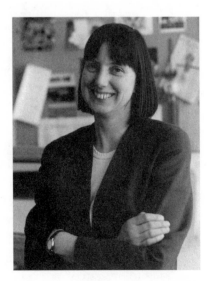

As a student she became deeply interested in infant feeding, with a special
concern for women who had problems breastfeeding. After qualifying as a
midwife, Mary worked with the Medical Research Council in Edinburgh. Here, as
part of an interdisciplinary team, she worked on research in breastfeeding, looking at the physiology of breastfeeding and at the problems that mothers and
babies have. As a researcher and practitioner, Mary was especially interested in
the views and experiences of women, and she found that little of this was
reflected in the research that was published in the field. She worked with many
breastfeeding mothers during this time, both in the hospital and in the community.

In 1982 she earned her doctorate in Edinburgh for her research in breastfeeding. She wanted to use her skills both to help women and to educate health care
practitioners in improving care for women and babies. After working as a
midwife in labor and delivery care in Oxford, England, Mary moved to Canada.
There she was associate professor in the School of Nursing at The University of
Lethbridge, Alberta, for three and a half years. She was also involved with the
grassroots midwifery movement in Canada and helped to found the Alberta
Association of Midwives, becoming its first spokesperson and Acting President.

In 1987, she returned to the United Kingdom and was appointed to a position
as Director of the Midwifery Research Programme at the National Perinatal
Epidemiology Unit in Oxford. She moved to Leeds in 1994 to take up her present
position, which includes developing a program of research in breastfeeding with
Dr. Mike Woolridge.

Mary had her first son, Jamie, in 1991 and her second, Calum, in 1993. Both
were born at home, where she was cared for by Chloe and another midwife
friend and colleague, Ethel. Jamie presented Mary (and Chloe!) with a wide range
of breastfeeding problems, including tongue tie and a colicky reaction whenever
Mary ate eggs. With lots of support, all eventually went well, but she now has a
much more intense understanding of breastfeeding problems, especially painful
feeding. Breastfeeding Calum was, by comparison, very straightforward; although
he resolutely refused any food or fluids except breastfeeding until he was over
8 months old. Her boys, now aged 6 and 7 1/2, are a constant source of joy, and
they continue to present new learning experiences on most days!

She travels internationally to teach and speak at conferences on midwifery and
breastfeeding, and continues to work with mothers and babies. Her aim is to
bring together the best of clinical research and clinical practice with women's
view of what they needs in maternity care.

"I have never felt comfortable with the idea that babies and families are
burdens to women that stand in the way of equality. The ability to bear a child
and to breastfeed are very powerful, creative aspects of being female. I want to

work toward an understanding of how women can have that power recognized and respected."

Chloe Fisher

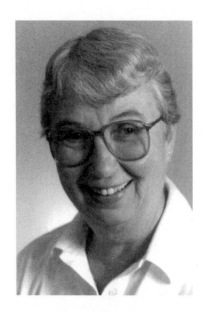

Chloe Fisher was a community midwife for more than thirty years. She was born in England in 1932, but spent the years during World War II in foster care in Canada because of the bombings in Britain. Her first training was as a nursery nurse; then she saw a birth, and discovered that she really wanted to be a midwife.

She did the first part of her midwifery training in Cambridge, England, where she worked in a small, midwife-run hospital maternity unit. She learned an enormous amount about breastfeeding there as a result of the good, continuous care given by the midwives. The second part of her training was done in a hospital in Oxford, England, where she saw the impact of artificial and restrictive practices on breastfeeding. When she did community midwifery, caring for women in their homes, she discovered her real love.

In her thirty-two years as a community midwife, Chloe has lost count of the number of mothers and babies for whom she has cared. She knows that by the early 1970s, she had delivered more than one thousand babies. In 1976 she became senior midwife for the Community Midwifery Service in Oxford. Her work in the community showed her that childbirth does not do well if rules are imposed, and also that feeding without rules or regulations prevents most breastfeeding problems.

In 1950 she read a pamphlet on feeding called *The Baby Who Does Not Conform to Rules*, which was important in shaping her own attitudes toward breastfeeding. "I've always felt babies should be treated with respect."

Chloe continues to teach midwives and physicians about helping mothers and babies form close relationships, of which breastfeeding is a special part. She now speaks throughout the United Kingdom and internationally and is an adviser to the International Lactation Consultant Association. She served as breastfeeding consultant to UNICEF in former Yugoslavia during the height of the conflict. She served as chair of the committee set up by the Royal College of Midwives in the United Kingdom to investigate the problems of breastfeeding. This committee produced a handbook for midwives, *Successful Breastfeeding*, which is a superb blend of research and clinical wisdom. In 1996, Chloe was awarded the MBE for services to infant health, a national recognition of her tremendous contribution to breastfeeding in the UK.

Chloe still works day to day with mothers and babies with breastfeeding problems. Her real love is helping mothers and babies get together. "This," she says, "has been the basis for all my work as a midwife."

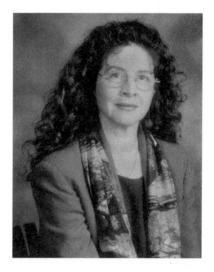

Suzanne Arms

Suzanne Arms, the third author, whose photographs also appear throughout this book, was born in New Jersey in 1944. She graduated from the University of Rochester, New York, in 1965 with honors in literature and a minor in anthropology. Afterward she moved to California, where she taught in day care centers, nursery schools, and Project Head Start, in urban, ghetto, and suburban settings. "I have always been committed to the healing of social ills, but I was an advocate for children long before I understood the relationship between children's and women's issues."

Having grown up during a time in the United States when both natural childbirth and breastfeeding were rare, Suzanne never saw a baby being breastfed until the age of twenty-six, when she was pregnant and living in a Northern California community in which both natural childbirth and breastfeeding were becoming common.

It was the birth of her daughter, Molly, in 1970 that inspired her to investigate modern childbirth practices. She researched, wrote, and did the photographs for *Immaculate Deception: A New Look at Women and Childbirth*. First published in 1975, it is no longer in print but is still considered a classic in its field. It is required reading in many college, nursing and midwifery courses. The New York Times named it a "Best Book of the Year". Her sequel, Immaculate Deception II: Myth, Magic and Birth (1997) is considered a current classic and includes a great deal of information on breastfeeding, bonding, and the sensitivity and awareness of newborns. She has also written To Love and Let Go (published in hardback in 1983, and now published in a much expanded and updated (1990) paperback edition as *Adoption: A Handful of Hope*). In 1994 she published Seasons of Change, her 7th book, focusing on the journey of pregnancy. In 1978 she made a childbirth education film, *Five Women, Five Births: A Film About Choices*, which has been widely used in birth classes since then. Her photographs have appeared in numerous books and publications. In 1999 she released her latest video, the first inspirational and educational video on natural normal birth and the midwifery model of care, called *Giving Birth: Challenges & Choices*.

After moving to Palo Alto, California, in 1976, she spearheaded the founding of The Birth Place, a nonprofit group that continues to operate a resource, information, and referral center on birth and parenting, and also a state-licensed childbirth center, near Stanford University. She is also a founding board member of Planetree, a national consumer health organization dedicated to improving hospital care and providing the public with access to medical information so they can be active participants in their own health and medical care. Planetree operates innovative health resource, information, and referral centers in San Francisco and other United States cities and a model hospital unit at Pacific Medical Center in San Francisco and at sites in other cities to assist communities and hospitals in making innovative changes.

As a writer, photographer and public speaker, she enjoys documenting the pioneering work of those who create positive models for change. Since 1970 she has been an active spokesperson for lay midwifery and home birth.

Suzanne and her husband, Dr Root Routledge, live in Durango, Colorado. Together they have formed a small company devoted to transforming birth and mother-baby practices, called Birthing The Future?. Their award-winning website, www.BirthingTheFuture.com, contains a wealth of information on maternity care and breastfeeding.

"Birth, infancy and early childhood experiences create the foundation for our lives. Not only does it affect our physical health and well-being, what we learn during this period of time forms the basis for who we become and how we feel about ourselves and our world. Breastfeeding is simply an integral part of that foundation."

Maggie Conroy

Maggie Conroy is an artist and illustrator who also founded a bookstore within an artists cooperative called the Artifactory, in Palo Alto, California. Today Maggie illustrates books, greeting cards, and birth announcements and also designs flyers.

She was born in Des Moines, Iowa, in 1956, attended Grandview College there, and then moved to Minneapolis and later to California, where she earned a master's degree in art therapy from the College of Notre Dame in 1983. Her first job was as an art therapist at Mills-Peninsula Hospital, near San Francisco, where she worked with preadolescent children with emotional difficulties, and with their parents. She also worked in several preschools in the San Francisco Bay area, including the Apple Childcare Center, which Apple Computer set up for the young children of its employees.

"As a preschool teacher I saw the concerns and challenges mothers faced in balancing child rearing, family, and work. In my work as a teacher and as an artist, I try to find ways to communicate understanding and support for the difficult balance women today must maintain between their roles as mother and as worker."

This book is a blend of all our experiences and backgrounds, and we are certain that no one of us could have written it without each of the others. Our goal has been to put into writing, photographs, and drawings the experience and knowledge we all have. Mary's writing skill, combined with academic knowledge and clinical understanding, Chloe's hands-on wisdom, Suzanne's understanding of women's needs, plus her extraordinary skill as a photographer and writer, together with Maggie's accurate and evocative drawings, made it possible to put together a book that is different from anything that has come before.

Learning about breastfeeding today, after so much knowledge and understanding has been lost through the years, it is not easy. We learned about breastfeeding by taking and working with mothers through many years (we have a total of seventy years' experience among us!), from personal experience of breastfeeding, and from reading about and studying the subject. We have also learned from each other in the course of writing. This book includes all of our approaches, and what it contains is what we all believe to be true.

Our plan was to write a clear, basic guide for women on how to get breastfeeding right and how to solve problems, with accurate information and pictures. We believe there is new and useful information in this book for everyone. If you find any parts especially helpful, or especially unhelpful, we would like to know. Please write to us, care of our publisher. This will help us improve the book in future editions.

Where to Find Help

YOU will find this list of addresses helpful if you want to contact groups that assist breastfeeding women. It is as up-to-date as we can make it. Some names and addresses may not be current by the time you read this book. We apologize if you have difficulty contacting any of them. Please let us know if this happens!

If you help to organize any of these groups and find that we have given an old address, please write to us in care of our publishers so we can update our list.

We know that there are many groups that help breastfeeding women that we have not listed for lack of space. The addresses listed here are to get you started. These groups will be able to put you in touch with local groups. If you know of a group in an area that we have not listed, please write to us.

Some of these are support groups for breast-feeding mothers, some are educational groups, and others are political pressure groups, such as International Baby Food Action Network (IBFAN). Any group will put you in touch with local breastfeeding support if they cannot give you help directly.

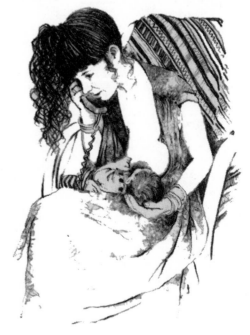

The list begins with international groups. Following these, the addresses are grouped by region or continent, and then broken down by country. Addresses for groups in the United Kingdom and the United States that assist parents of babies with special needs follow the general list. Closing this section are national and international addresses for companies you can write or call for information on renting or purchasing breast pumps.

International

International Childbirth Education
  Association
PO Box 20048
Minneapolis, MN 55420
USA
Tel. + 1 (612) 854 8660
Fax + 1 (612) 854 8772
Email: info@icea.org
Website: http://www.icea.org

The IBLCE International Office:
Serving the America and sub-Saharan Africa:
IBLCE
PO Box 2348
Falls Church, VA 22042-0348 USA
Tel: + 1 (703) 560-7330
Fax: + 1 (703) 560-7332
Email: iblce@erols.com
Website: http://www.iblce.org/

IBLCE Regional Office in Australia:
Serving Asia and the South Pacific:
Ros Escott, Regional Administrator
PO Box 13,
South Hobart, TAS 7004
AUSTRALIA
Tel: + 61 (03) 6223-8445
Fax: + 61 (03) 6223-8665
Email: escoa@mpx.com.au

IBLCE Regional Office in Germany:
Serving Europe, the Middle East, and North
  Africa
Erika Nehlsen, Regional Administrator
Sudhang 4,
32457 Porta Westfalica
GERMANY
Tel: + 49 (0571) 798-9025
Fax: + 49 (0571) 76921

International Confederation of Midwives
  (ICM)
Eisenhouwerlaan 138
2517 KN
The Hague
The Netherlands

International Lactation Consultant
  Association (ILCA)
Suite 201
4101 Lake Boone Trail
Raleigh, NC 27607
Tel: + 1 (919) 787-5181
Fax: + 1 (919) 787-4916
Email: ilca@erols.com
Website: http://www.ilca.org/

La Leche League International
1400 N. Meacham Rd.
Schaumburg, IL 60173-4048
USA
Tel: + 1 (847) 519-7730
Fax: + 1 (847) 519-0035
Email: lllhq@llli.org
Website: http://www.lalecheleague.org/
(Or for languages other than English)
    http://www.lalecheleague.org/LLLIlang.html
See also under individual countries
    (LLL = La Leche League).

World Alliance for Breastfeeding Action
  (WABA)
PO Box 1200
10850 Penang
Malaysia.
Tel: + 60 (4) 658 4816
Fax: + 60 (4) 657 2655
Email: secr@waba.po.my
Website: http://www.elogica.com.br/waba

UNICEF
Margaret Kyenkya
NGO Liaison
UNICEF H8F, 3 UN Plaza,
New York NY 10017.
Tel: +1 (212) 326 7000
Website: http://www.unicef.org

Teaching Aids at Low Cost (TALC)
P.O. Box 49, St. Albans
Herts AL1 4AX, United Kingdom
Tel: (01727) 853 869
Fax: (01727) 846 852

IBFAN
Website: http://www.gn.apc.org/ibfan/
for other details see Regional offices

Africa

IBFAN Africa
Centrepoint
Cnr of Tin and Walker Streets
Mbabane
Swaziland
Tel: (+268) 45006 and 43228
Fax: (+268) 40546
Email: PKisanga@realnet.co.sz

IBFAN Afrique Francophone
01 BP 6287
Ouagadougou 01
Burkina Faso
Ph: (+226) 314 109
Fax: (+226) 300 968

Burkina [+226]

Association Pour la Promotion de
   l'Alimentation Infantile Burkinabe (APAIB)
01 BP 6287
Ouagadougou 01, Burkina Faso
Tel: 3141-09

IBFAN Burkina
213 Avenue Kadiogo
01 BP. 1776
Ouagadougou 01, Burkina Faso
Tel: 303804
Fax: 303888

Botswana [+267]

Breastfeeding Promotion Group
P.O. Box 992
Gabarone, Botswana
*unknown to International Directory
   Assistance

Egypt [+20]

Egyptian Society of Breast Milk Friends
Al-Hussein University Hospital
Al-Azhar
Cairo, Egypt
Tel: (02) 915761

Ghana [+233]

Developing Countries Health Radio Network
PO Box 15902
Accra, Ghana
*unknown to International Directory
   Assistance

Ivory Coast [+225]

Institut National de Sante Publique
Boite Postal V47
Abidjan, Cote d'Ivoire
Tel: 22 44 04

Kenya [+254]

Breastfeeding Information
Chiromo Rd.
PO Box 59436
Nairobi
Ph: (02) 749 899
Fax: (02) 443 241

Kenya Food and Nutrition Action Network
(KEFAN)
P. O. Box 47639
Nairobi
Tel: (02) 561766

Mauritius [+230]

Mauritian Action for the Promotion of
Breastfeeding and Infant Nutrition
(MAPBIN)
PO Box 1134
Port-Louis, ile Maurice
Tel: 211 4433
Fax: 211 4436
Email: icpmapbi@intnet.mu

Sierra Leone [+232]

Sierra Leone Infant Feeding Action Group
(SLIFAG)
Dr. Elvira Faux-During, Vice-president
PMB 22, Freetown
Tel: (022) 225738 or 223651
Fax: (022) 224439

South Africa [+27]

SALCA (Southern African Lactation
Consultants Association),
PO Box 1227,
Roosevelt Park, 2129
Fax/answering machine: (011) 888-1086
Email: lynn@mod.co.za

NABA (National Alliance for Breastfeeding
Action, South Africa),
PO Box 222,
Auckland Park, 2006.

LLL-SA
PO Box 10153,
Aston Manor, 1630.
Tel/Fax: (031) 309 1801
Email: pc16@pixie.co.za
Website: http://www.prairienet.org/llli/
WebSouthAfrica.html

Breastfeeding Association of South Africa
(BFA-SA),
(mother-to-mother phone counselling)
PO Box 4055,
Old Oak Village, 7537.
Tel: (021) 646-8363

Swaziland [+268]

Swaziland Infant Nutrition Action Network
(SINAN)
PO Box 1032
Mbabane
Tel: 45006
Fax: 40546

Tanzania [+255]

Tanzania Food and Nutrition Centre (TFNC)
P.O. Box 977
Dar Es Salaam
Tel: (051) 29621 or 29622 or 29623
Fax: (051) 28951

Uganda [+256]

Safe Motherhood Initiative Uganda
P.O. Box 1191
Kampala
Tel: (041) 23 57 91
Fax: (041) 23 07 84

The Uganda Lactation Management and
Education Team (ULMET)
Makerere University
P. O. Box 10202
Kampala
Tel:

Zimbabwe [+263]

Southern African Lactation Consultants
Association (in Zimbabwe)
10 Camberwell Close
Borrowdale
Harare
Tel: (04) 883500
Fax: (04) 498870
Email: mhc@harare.iafrica.com

LLL Zimbabwe
P O Box RVL48
Runiville, Harare
Tel/fax: (04) 495618; also (04) 497051
Email: tna@harare.iafrica.com
Website:
  http://www.prairienet.org/llli/WebZimbabw
  e.html

Asia

IBFAN Asia
c/o Citizens' Alliance for Consumer
  Protection
KPO Box 411
Seoul 110-062, Korea
Tel: +82 (02) 738 2555
Fax: +82 (02) 736 5514
Email: cacpk@chollian.dacom.co.kr

South Asia Breastfeeding Promotion
  Network of India (BPNI)
P O Box 10551, BP-33
Pitampura Delhi 110 034, India
Tel/Fax: +91 (011) 721 9606
OR
Phone: (91-11) 7211435
Fax: (91-11) 7134787

Bangladesh [+880]

ODA-NGO Project
House 10, Road 5
Dhanmodi R/A
Dhaka

China [+86]

Shanghai Medical University
Box 209
Shanghai
(just research)

Hong Kong [+852]

LLL Hong Kong
Tel: 2548-7636
Fax: 2548-8202
Email: Judith_Trudel@compuserve.com
Website: http://www.prairienet.org/llli/
  WebHongKong.html

Indonesia [+62]

Badan Kerja Peningkatan Penggunaan Air
Susu Ibu
Yasia Office
Bagian Ilmu Kesehatan Anak (GE-IKA), FKUI-
  RSCM
JL Salemba 6 - Jakarta Pusat

Malaysia [+60]

IBFAN Penang
PO Box 19
10700 Penang
OR
26 N Jalan Mafjid Negeri Jelutong
Ph: (04) 656 9799
Fax: (04) 657 7291

Parenting Concepts
Sdn Bhd., 2776B, 1st floor,
Jalan Cangkat Permata,
Taman Permata, 53300 Kuala Lumpur.
Tel: (03) 405 3872/3;
Fax: (03) 406 8914.
Email: tasmim@tm.net.my

PPPIM (Breastfeeding Advisory Association
  of Malaysia),
25A, Jalan Kampong Pandan
53100 Kuala Lumpur

Philippines [+63]

Aarugaan
42-A Maalalahanin St.
Teacher's Village,
Quezon City
Phone: (02) 922-5189 or 921-7080

Balikatan at Ugnayang Naglalayong Sumagip
   sa Sanggol (BUNSO)
#5 Basilan Road, Philam Homes
Quezon City
Tel: (02) 99-12-17
Fax: (02) 921-2690 (Attn: Child Manila)

Singapore [+65]

Breastfeeding Mothers Support Group(s)
No. 8 Robinson Road #06-00
COSCO Building
Singapore 048544
Counselling Hotline: 339-3558
Email: bmsg@iname.com
Website:
   http://members.tripod.com/~bmsg/

Caribbean

Caribbean Food & Nutrition Institute (CFNI)
University of the West Indies Campus
P.O. Box 140
Kingston 7, Jamaica

Dominican Republic [+1]

LLL of the Dominican Republic
Yanet Olivares de Saiz
Postal address: ASC # 3217, 5635 N.W. 74
   Ave., MIAMI FL, 33166
Home address: Miguel Angel Monclús #356,
   Residencial KJ, Apt. C4, Mirador
Norte, Santo Domingo, República
   Dominicana
Tel: (809) 530 0029
Email: m.saiz@codetel.net.do
Website: http://www.prairienet.org/llli/
   WebDominica.html

Dutch Antilles [+59]

Fundashion Leche di Mama
#2 Concientiesteeg
Curacao
Tel: (99) 462 5852

Trinidad [+1]

The Informative Breast Feeding Service
   (TIBS)
8 Rust Street, St. Clair
Port-of-Spain, Trinidad, W.I.
Tel: (868) 628-8234
Fax: (868) 681-269

Central and South America

Grupo Origem (WABA Brazil, IBFAN
   Regional)
Av. Beira Mar, 3661 lj.18
Casa Caiada
Olinda PE
Tel: +55 (081) 4327701
Fax: +55 (081) 4327701
Email: origem@elogica.com.br
Website:
   http://bbs.elogica.com.br/aleitamento

Regional Resource Centre - see under
   Fundacion Lacmat (Argentina)

IBFAN Latin America
25 Ave. 2-70
Zona 7
Residencias Altamira
Ciudad de Guatemala
Guatemala
Email: ruth.arango@starnet.net.gt
OR
International Baby Food Action Network
   (IBFAN) Latin America
Amamanta
Apartado Postal No. 80273
Caracas 1080, Venezuela
Tel: (58-2)
Fax: (58-2) 977 0476

CEPREN - Centro de Promocion de Estudios
en Nutricion
Av. Pardo, 1335 OF.302
Lima-18 Peru
Tel: +51 (01) 445-1978
Fax: +51 (01) 241-6205
Email: cepren@amauta.rcp.net.pe

Argentina [+54]

Fundacion Lacmat - IBFAN Argentina
C. C. 27, Suc. S. A. de Padua
(1718) Buenos Aires
Tel/Fax: (020) 850 687
Email: fundalac@yahoo.com
(or for the Regional Resource Centre) docu-
lac@yahoo.com
Website: http://www.fmed.uba.ar/mspba/fun-
dalac/
(or for IBFAN Argentina)
http://www.fmed.uba.ar/mspba/ibfarg/

Asociacion Ayuda Materna Nunu
Guemos 2001, Florida
Buenos Aires (1602)
Tel/Fax: (01) 791 9490

Belize [+501]

Breast is Best League (BIB)
P.O. Box 1208
Belize City
Tel: (02) 77398

Bolivia [+591]

Comite Tecnico de Apoyo a la Lactancia
Materna (COTALMA)
Av. Arce 2105 Edificio Venus 5o piso,
Dpto 5B.
La Paz
Tel/Fax: (02) 350304

La Liga de la Leche en Bolivia (LLL Bolivia)
Casilla 10077
La Paz
Phone: (02) 791699

Brazil [+55]

IBFAN Brazil
Rua Santo Antonio 590
2 Andar
Sao Paulo 01314-000
Tel/Fax: (011) 832 6889

Pastoral da Criança (Pastoral of the Child)
Rua Pasteur, 279
80250-902 Curitiba, Paraná
Tel: (041) 322-0704
Fax: (041) 224-6986
Email: pastcri@rebidia.org.br
Website: http://www.rebidia.org.br/

Clínica Interdisciplinar de Apoio à
Amamentação
Rua Visconde de Pirajá, 414 / 1019
22410-002 Rio de Janeiro - RJ
Brasil
Tel: (021) 5228897
Fax: (021) 5229680
Email: ibfanrio@ax.apc.org
Website:
http://www.alternex.com.br/ ~ ibfanrio/clini
ca4.htm

Programa de Aleitamento Materno
(PROAMA)
Central de Informacoes de Maes para a
Amamentacao (CIMAMA)
Rua Comendador Araujo, 252 3o andar -.
sala 45
80420-000 Curitiba, PR
Tel: (041) 322-6533/108 or 322-1515/131
Fax: (041) 225-4373

Chile [+56]

Liga Chilena de la Lactancia Materna
Casilla 90 T. Providencia
Santiago

Colombia [+ 57]

LLL Colombia
Apartado Aereo 94764,
Bogota
Tel: (571) 616-2500 o (571) 616-1300 -
  Código: Liga de la Leche- (es un Beeper)
Email: mjposada@hotmail.com
Website: http://www.prairienet.org/llli/
  WebColombia.html

Costa Rica [+ 506]

Comision Nacional de Lactancia Materna
Tres Rios
Cartago
Tel: 79-99-11
Fax: 79-55-46

Ecuador [+ 593]

Centro Medico de Orientacion y
  Planificacion Familiar (CEMOPLAF)
Casilla 3549
Quito
Tel: (02) 518-251
Fax: (02) 582-435

Guatemala [+ 502]

Comision Nacional de Promocion de la
  Lactancia Materna (CONAPLAM)
6a Av. 0-60, Torre Profesional I, 8o Nivel Of
  804, Gran Centro Comercial Z. 4.
Guatemala City
Tel: (02) 315892 or 351633 or 351928
Fax: (02) 351947

Honduras [+ 504]

Asociacion Hondurena de Lactancia Materna
  (AHLACMA)
Apartado Postal No. 3465
Tegucigalpa
Tel: 327 287

Unidad de Lactancia Materna, Hospital
  Escuela, Ministerio de Salud Publica
4to Piso B.M.I., Boulevard Estadio - Suyapa
Tegucigalpa
Phone: 322 322, ext. 336

Mexico [+ 52]

Centro de Promocion y Proteccion de la
  Lactancia Materna (CEPPLAM)
Apartado Postal No. 30
Chiapa de Corzo, Chiapas C.P. 29160
Tel/Fax: (0968) 6 06 41

La Liga de la Leche de Mexico A.C.
Francisco Petarca 223-402, Col Polanco
C. P. 11560
Mexico City, D.F.
Phone: (05) 531 28 03

Peru [+ 51]

LLL Peru
c/o Claudia Jimenez
Embajada de Mexico
Av. Santa Cruz #330
Col San Isidro
Lima
Email: jimenez@amauta.rcp.net.pe
Website: http://www.prairienet.org/llli/
  WebPeru.html

Uruguay [+ 598]

PRAIL-LAC
c/o CLAP/PAHO
Hospital de Clinicas, Piso 16
Montevideo
Phone: (02) 472-929
Fax: (02) 472-593

Europe

IBFAN EUROPE (Also GIFA, a Swiss group)
PO Box 157
1211 Geneva 19
Switzerland
Ph: +41 (022) 798 9164
Fax: +41 (022) 798 4443
Email: philipec@iprolink.ch

Societe Europeenne pour le Soutien de
l'Allaitement Maternel (SESAM)
8, rue de Jarente
75004 Paris, France
Tel: (01) 42 77 74 37
Fax: (01) 42 74 56 62

Albania [+355]

Albanian Group for the Protection and Pro-
motion of Breastfeeding (IBFAN member)
c/o Women's Center
PO Box 2418
Tirana
Tel/Fax: (042) 23693
Fax: (042) 35855
Email: ibfan@women-center.tirana.al

Armenia [+374]

"Confidence" c/o ICU
PO Box 586
Yerevan 375010
Tel: (02) 341 583
Fax: (02) 151 957
Email: c/o ICU: icu@arminco.com

Austria [+43]

LLL Austria
Postfach, A-6240 Rattenberg
Tel/Fax: (01) 876 5827
Email: oliv@telecom.at
Website: http://www.telecom.at/lalecheliga/

Verband der Still- und Laktationsberaterin-
nen Osterreichs IBCLC (VSLOE)
(Austrian Association of Lactation
Consultants IBCLC),
c/o Anne-Marie Kern,
Lindenstrasse 20,
A-2362 Biedermannsdorf.
Tel/Fax: (022) 367 2336
Email: e.kern@online.edvg.co.at

Belgium [+32]

VBBB: Vereniging voor Begeleiding en
Bevordering van Borstvoeding
(Organisation for Supporting and Promoting
Breastfeeding)
Cardijnstraat 36
2910 Essen
Tel: (03) 677 1318
Fax: (03) 677 1748
Email: vbbb@village.uunet.be
Website: http://www.omnicon.be/vbbb/
vbbb.htm

Brussels Childbirth Trust (English and
French speaking)
Rue Auguste Lambiotte 62
1030 Schaerbeek
Tel: (02) 215 3377

Bosnia Herzegovina [+387]

Breastfeeding Advancement Group
Kotromaniceva 5/111 FBH
71000 Sarajevo
Tel/Fax: (071) 521 294

Bulgaria [+359]

"Women and mothers against violence" -
(IBFAN Bulgaria)
Sofia 1233
"Strouga" str., Bl. 40 A, entr. "Á"
Tel: (02) 32 60 88
Fax: (02) 45 30 48
Email: ubs_bulgaria@yahoo.com

Croatia [+385]

Croatian Breastfeeding Promotion Group
Horvatovac 67
10000 Zagreb
Tel/Fax: (01) 455 7071
Email: hupd@zg.tel.hr

Czech Republic [+42]

ANIMA (IBFAN Prague)
c/o 3rd Medical School
Charles University
Ruská 87
100 00 Prague 10
Tel: (02) 671 023 40
Fax: (02) 673 118 12 (Att: Dagmar
    Schneidrova)
Email: c/o Dagmar.Schneidrova@lf3.cuni.cz

Finland [+358]

Raittiuden Ystövöt
c/o RY/ETRA
Annankatu 29 A9
00100 Helsinki
Tel: (09) 694 4177
Fax: (09) 694 4407
Email: ritva.kuusisto@raitis.fi

France [+33]

Action pour l'Allaitement
BP 42
67044 STRASBOURG Cedex
Tel: (0388) 611 747
Fax: (0388) 606 937
Email: camwal@imaginet.fr
Website: http://web.superb.net/apastras/

Association Francaise des Consultants en
    Lactation
French Association of Lactation Consultants,
c/o Lea Cohen (English and French spoken),
116 Rue du General Leclerc,
78420 Carrieres sur Seine
Tel: (01) 3968 1081

LLL France,
BP 18, l'Etang la Ville,
France 78620
Tel: (01) 39 584 584
Website: http://www.lllfrance.org/

Information pour l'Allaitement (IPA)
52, rue Sully
F-69006 LYON
Tel/Fax: (04) 78 93 02 08
Email: nathalie.roques@wanadoo.fr
Website: http://perso.wanadoo.fr/ipa/

Solidarilait,
Centre Puercultrice,
26 Bvd. Brune,
F-75014 Paris.
Tel. 01 40 44 70 70 (Answering Machine)

Centre de Formation et de Documentation
    sur l'Allaitement Maternel (CFDAM),
Maternité 76170 Lillebonne;
Tel: (02) 35 96 39 24.

Co-naître,
Institut de Formation,
Secrétariat des Formations,
L'Escandihado, route de la Bonde,
84120 Pertuis
Tel: (06) 09 52 53 79 from 1pm to 6pm
Fax/answering machine: (04) 90 79 58 21.

Georgia [+995]

Child Health Nutrition Fund
"CLARITAS"
TEVS district, 11 m/r
Tbilisi 380091
Tel: (032) 943 448
Fax: (032) 940 009
Email: nemsadze@tmgph.kheta.ge

Germany [+49]

Arbeitsgemeinschaft Freier Stillgruppen
  (AFS)
Gertraudgasse 4R
97070 Würzburg
Tel: (0931) 573 493
Fax: (0931) 573 494
Email: AFS-Stillgruppen@t-online.de
Website: http://www.stillen.org/

Bund Deutscher Laktationsberaterinnen
(German Association of Lactation
  Consultants)
Elke Sporleder,
D-30457 Hannover,
Delpweg 14.
Tel: (0511) 467 164;
Fax: (0511) 465 906
Email: info@stillen.de
Website: http://www.stillen.de

LLL Deutschland e.V.
Postfach 650096
81214 München
Tel/fax: 06851-2524
Email: lll.d@bigfoot.com
Website: http://www.carpeNet.de/LaLeche/

Greece [+30]

Greek Association of Lactation Consultants,
Tel: (031) 656 703

Hungary [+36]

Hungarian Association for Breastfeeding
55 Margit Krt.
Budapest 1024
Tel/Fax: (01) 316 6762
(Alternative contact details:
  c/o Dr. Katalin Sarlai (President)
  21 Csalogany
  Budapest 1027
  Tel: (01) 201 7849)
Email: hab@c3.hu
Website: http://www.c3.hu/ ~ hab

Ireland [+353]

Association of Lactation Consultants in
  Ireland (ALCI),
c/o Dr. Carol Campbell,
Clinical Medical Officer in Community
  Paediatrics,
Deerpark,
37 Ballyquin Rd.,
Limavady,
Co. Derry BT49 9EY,
Northern Ireland
Tel: (01504) 762 321
Fax: (01504) 611 254
Email: ccampbell@btinternet.com

Baby Milk Action
c/o 10 Upper Camden St.
Dublin 2
Tel: (01) 462 2026
Fax: (01) 662 5493
Email: babymilkaction@tinet.ie

La Leche League Ireland
LLL Ireland is listed in all local telephone
  directories - check there for contact details
  of your nearest group.
Website: http://homepage.tinet.ie/ ~ laleche-
  league/index.html

Israel [+972]

Israel Lactation Consultants (Evi Adams),
16 Masada St., Ashdod.
Email: evadams@ibm.net

Italy [+39]

Breastfeeding Support Group
Burlo Garofolo Children's Hospital of Trieste
Via dell'Isteria 65 1
Trieste 34137
Tel: (040) 378 5236
Fax: (040) 378 5402
Email: bih@burlo.trieste.it
Website: http://www.burlo.trieste.it

LLL Italia
Casella Postale 1368,
20100 Milano
Website: http://www.lalecheleague.org/Lang/
    LangItaliano.html

Kazakhstan [+7]

JAN SABI
66 Klochkov Str.
480008 Almaty
Tel: (03272) 422 543
Fax: (03272) 429 203
Email: zaure@nutrit1.almaty.kz

Latvia [+371]

LKEVAB
16 Dzierciema Str.
LV 1007 Riga
Tel: 253 6189
Fax: 782 8155
Email: iranka@lanet.lv

Lithuania [+370]

Lithuanian Breastfeeding Support Society
Eiveniu 4 - 115
Kaunas 3007
Tel: (07) 794 736
Fax: (07) 796 498
Email: SOCPED@KMA.LT

Luxembourg [+352]

Initiativ Liewensufank a.s.b.l.
20 rue de Contern
L-5955 Itzig
Tel: 36 05 98
Fax: 36 61 34
Email: maryse.lehners@ci.educ.lu
Website: www.liewensufank.lu

Malta [+356]

Association of Breastfeeding Counsellors
175, P.P. Bezzina Str.
Ta'Zwejt
San Gwann SGN 09
Tel: 371 700
Fax: 250 052
Email: lizc@global.net.mt

Netherlands [+31]

Vereniging Borstvoeding Natuurlijk,
Postbus 119, 3960 BC Wijk bij Duurstede.
Tel: 0343 576626;
Email: borstvoeding_natuurlijk@knoware.nl
Website: http://utopia.knoware.nl/users/vbn

LLL Nederland
Postbus 212
4300 AE Zierikzee
Tel: 0111- 413189
Postbank 5391280
Email: hcats@xs4all.nl
Website: http://www.xs4all.nl/ ~ llln/

Nederlandse Verenigung van
    Lactatiekundigen (NVL),
Postbus 5243,
2701 GE Zoetermeer.
OR: W. Arondeusstraat 10
    4333 DA Middelburg
Tel: 793 213 693
OR:118 615 041
Fax: 793 290 061

Wemos Foundation (Working Group on
    Health and Development Issues)
P.O. Box 1693
1000 BR Amsterdam
Tel: (020) 4688388
Fax: (020) 4686008
Email: wemos@wemos.nl
Website: http://www.wemos.nl

Norway [+47]

Ammehjelpen, and AHIG, c/o
  Ammehjelpens sekretariat,
2423 Østby, Norway.
Berit Marie Oyeshaug (secretary/
  administrator).
Tel: 6245 5251
Fax: 6245 5105
Email: ammehjelpen@c2i.net

Ammefagradet (Breastfeeding resource
  group)
c/o Grø Nylander,
Kvinneklinikken, Rikshospitalet,
N-0027 Oslo.
Tel: 2286 9215;
Fax: 2286 9235.

Poland [+48]

Department of Breastfeeding Promotion
Institute of Mother and Child
ul. Kasprzaka 17A
01-211 Warszawa
Tel: (022) 632 3674
Fax: (022) 632 9454

Slovakia [+42]

Pro Vita
Univ. Children's Hospital
Dpt. Of Pediatrics
Limbova 1
833 40 Bratislava
Tel: (017) 760 619
Fax: (017) 375 752
Email: provita@gtinet.sk

Spain [+34]

ACPAM (Associació Catalana Pro Alletament
  Matern) (resource distributors)
C/ Benet Mercadé 9, bajos
08012 Barcelona
Tel/Fax: (093) 337 4787
Email: acpam@pangea.org

La Liga de la Leche de Euskadi
Apdo 5044
48080 Bilbao
Tel: (94) 423 01 36
   (94) 427 03 53
   (94) 328 63 59

LLL-Madrid
(91) 734 91 34
(91) 663 99 46
(91) 328 29 00

LLL-Cataluña
(908) 826 50 24

LLL-Andalusia
(95) 232 39 05

Asociacion de Madres Via Lactea
(Grupo de apoyo a la lactancia)
C/ Terminillo, 60-64, 2° IZDA.
50017 ZARAGOZA
Tel/Fax: (0976) 349 920
Email: mblazq2@acacia.pntic.mec.es
   juberias@posta.unizar.es

Sweden [+46]

Amningshjälpen
Box 54, 274 03 Rydsgård
Tel/Fax: (0411) 44 333
Email: rikskontor@amningshjalpen.se
Website: http://www.amningshjalpen.se/

Svenska Amningsinstitutet,
Kronhusgatan 2 E, 1tr,
Göteborg, S-41113
Tel: (031) 774 2870
Fax: (031) 152 819
Email: britta.heydenberg@tripnet.se

Switzerland [+41]

BSS Berufsverband Schweizerischer
   Stillberaterinnen
(Swiss Association of Lactation Consultants)
P.O.Box 686, Office CH-3000 Bern 25
Phone (041) 671 01 73
Fax (041) 671 01 71
Email: BSS.Geschaeftsstelle@gmx.net
Website: under construction at time of going
   to press.

LLL Schweiz
Postfach 197
8053 Zürich
Tel/Fax: (052) 243 11 44
Website: http://www.ajm.ch/lllref.html

United Kingdom [+44]

Association of Breastfeeding Mothers
PO Box 207
Bridgewater TA6 7YT
Tel: 020 7813 1481
Fax: 0117 966 1788
Email: abm@clara.net
Website: http://home.clara.net/abm/

Baby Milk Action (BMA)
23 St. Andrew's St.
Cambridge CB2 3AX
Tel: 01223 464420
Fax: 01223 464417
Email: babymilkacti@gn.apc.org
Website: http://www.gn.apc.org/babymilk/

Breastfeeding Network,
PO Box 11126,
Paisley PA2 8YB,
Scotland.
Tel: 0870 900 8787 (This will put the caller
   straight through to her nearest
   Breastfeeding
Network Supporter at national call rates)
Email: broadfoot@btinternet.com

Breastfeeding Promotion Group
& Joint Breastfeeding Initiative
National Childbirth Trust (NCT)
Alexandra House
Oldham Terrace
Acton, London W3 6NH
Tel: 020 8992 8637
Fax: 020 8992 5929

Healthlink Worldwide (formerly AHRTAG)
29-35 Farringdon Rd.,
London EC1 M3JB;
tel: 020 7242 0606;
Fax: 020 7242 0041.
E-mail: info@healthlink.org.uk
Website: http://www.poptel.org.uk/ahrtag

Lactation Consultants of Great Britain
   (LCGB),
111 Pilgrim's Way, Kemsing,
Seven Oaks, Kent TN15 6TE.
Tel: (01585) 493873

LLL Great Britain,
PO Box 29, Westbridgford
Nottingham NG2 7NP
Tel: 020 7242 1278.
http://www.stargate.co.uk/lllgb/

MIDIRS,
9 Elmdale Rd.
Clifton, Bristol BS8 1SL
Tel: 0117 925 1791
Freecall inside UK: 0800 581009
Fax: 0117 925 1792
Email: midirs@dial.pipex.com
Website: http://www.midirs.org/

Royal College of Midwives,
15 Mansfield St,
London WIM OBE
Tel: (020) 7872 5100
Fax: (020) 7312 3536

North America

Infant Feeding Action (INFACT) Canada
    (IBFAN North America)
6 Trinity Square, Toronto, Canada. M5G 1B1
Tel: +1 (416) 595-9819
Fax: +1 (416) 591-9355
Email: infact@ftn.net
Website: http://www.infactcanada.ca

Canada [+1]

LLL Canada
Freecall: 1-800-665-4324

LLL Canada Français
Case postale 874
Ville Saint-Laurent.
Québec Canada H4L 4W3
Tel (Montréal): (514) 525-3243
Tel (Quebec): (418) 653-2349
Website: http://www.prairienet.org/llli/
    WebLLLCF.html

USA [+1]

National Alliance for Breastfeeding Advocacy
    (NABA)
c/o Marsha Walker,
Office of Educational Services
254 Conant Rd.
Weston, MA 02493-1756
Tel: (781) 893-3553
Fax: (781) 893-8608
Email: Marshalact@aol.com
Website: http://members.aol.com/
    marshalact/Naba/

Breastfeeding Support Consultants (BSC)
228 Park Lane,
Chalfont PA 18914-3135
Tel: (215) 822 1281
Fax: (215) 997 7879
Email: info@bsccenter.org
Website: http://www.bsccenter.org/

Bright Future Lactation Resource Centre,
6540 Cedarview Court,
Dayton, Ohio 45459;
Tel: 937 438 9458;
Fax 937 438 3229;
Email: lindaj@bflrc.com
Website: http://www.bflrc.com

Wellstart San Diego Lactation Program
4062 First Ave.
San Diego CA 92103
Tel: (619) 295 5192
Fax: (619) 294 7787
Email: inquiry@wellstart.org
Website: http://www.wellstart.org/

Women's International Public Health
    Network (WIPHN)
7100 Oak Forest Lane
Bethesda MD 20817
Tel: (301) 469 9210
Fax: (301) 469 8423
Email: wiphn@erols.com

South Pacific

Australia [+61]

Nursing Mothers' Association of Australia
    (NMAA)
(NMAA runs the Lactation Resource Centre,
    an international library of breastfeeding
    information - see below))
P.O. Box 4000
Glen Iris, Victoria 3146
Tel: (03) 9885 0855
Fax: (03) 9885 0866
Email: nursingm@vicnet.net.au
Website: http://www.nmaa.asn.au
Lactation Resource Centre
For mailing address, phone and fax see
    NMAA
Email: lrc@vicnet.net.au
Website: http://www.nmaa.asn.au/lrc

ALCA (Australian Lactation Consultants'
  Association)
PO Box 192,
Mawson ACT 2607
Tel/Fax: (02) 6290 1920
Email: alcagalaxy@interact.net.au

Fiji [+679]

National Food and Nutrition Committee
P.O. Box 2450, Suva
Phone: 25834 or 313055

New Zealand [+64]

NZ Lactation Consultants' Association,
Po Box 29-279,
Christchurch, NZ

LLL New Zealand,
Box 13383,
Johnsonville, Wellington 4
Tel: (04) 478-1315
Email: lllnz@clear.net.nz
Website: http://www.lalecheleague.org/
  LLLNZ/

**Many of the organizations listed on the
previous pages will give you information
about pumps and pump hire. You can
also try the following organisations:**

Avent America Inc. Tel (800) 542 8367.
  www.aventamerica.com

Egnell Ameda Ltd. Unit 2, Belevedere
  Trading Estate, Taunton, Somerset TA1
  1BH. Tel 01823 336362

Medela (UK), Expressions Breastfeeding,
  CMS House, Basford Lane, Leakbrook,
  Leak, Staffordshire ST13 7DP. Tel 01538
  386650

Medela (USA) www.medela.com

National Childbirth Trust/Egnell breast pump
  hire (UK) 0122252 655419

Books You Might Find Helpful

*S*OME of you may like more detail on specific aspects of breastfeeding that we have been able to provide in this book. This is a short list of books that you might find helpful.

Balancing Acts: On Being a Mother, Katherine Gleve, ed. (London: Virago, 1989). If you want to know how other women feel about being mothers and the challenges of mothering in Western culture, this book will interest you. It is a collection of women's accounts, telling their experiences and feelings.

Breastfeeding Matters, Maureen Minchin (Melbourne, Australia: Alma Publications, 1998). This book is a good review of the practical problems and the politics of infant feeding. It is well referenced and full of facts on all aspects of breastfeeding: nutrition, allergies, culture, and practical aspects such as positioning. Available in North America through Birth and Life Bookstore, P.O. Box 70625,

Seattle, WA 98107 (telephone: (206) 789-4444); in the United Kingdom through the National Childbirth Trust (see address in "Where to Find Help"); or direct from Alma Publications, 5 St. George's Rd., Armadale, Victoria, Australia.

Breastfeeding special care babies. Sandra Lang. W.B. Saunders Co. 1996. A helpful book about breastfeeding babies who are in special care units.

Cleft Lip and Palate; a parents' guide. Cleft Lip and Palate Association/Kings Fund, Royal College of Surgeons, London. Available from Cleft Lip and Palate Association, 138 Buckingham Palace Road, London SW1W 9FA. A helpful guide to feeding a baby who has a cleft lip or palate.

Crying Babies, Sleepless Nights, Sandy Jones (New York: Harvard Common Press, 1994). Dedicated to "all the mothers who are reading this book at 4 a.m., and to all the babies who long not to have to cry anymore." This book will be a good, practical support for anyone with an inconsolable baby.

Drugs, Vitamins, Minerals in Pregnancy, Ann K. Henry and Jil Feldhausen (Tucson, AZ: Fisher Books, 1989). This is an easy-to-read book listing the commonly used drugs or medications and their possible side effects when taken during pregnancy or lactation. It can be obtained directly through Fisher Books, P.O. Box 38040, Tucson, AZ 85740-8040, U.S.A.

Hi Mom! Hi Dad!: The First Twelve Months of Parenthood (101 cartoons). Lynn Johnston (Toronto: Stoddart Publishing Co., 1985). These wonderful cartoons will entertain you and at the same time reassure you that life with a new baby is a mixture of joy, frustration, and exhaustion. An important book to keep you balanced and laughing with your new baby around.

Medications and Mothers Milk, Thomas Hale, Pharmasoft Medical Publishing, 1998-1999. Web site adress: http://neonatal.ttuhsc.edu/lact/. This book gives information about the safety of medications taken while breastfeeding.

Nursing Mother's Companion, Kathleen Huggins (Boston: Souvenir Press, 1983). We recommend this book's section on working

outside the home and breastfeeding called "Traveling Together, Being Apart." It gives practical suggestions on how to breastfeed while being separated from your baby, and summarizes the types of breast pumps that are available, discussing the advantages and disadvantages of each.

The Politics of Breastfeeding, Gabrielle Palmer (Rivers Oram Press/Pandora List, 1993). An excellent discussion for the problems women face today. It covers political, economic, and cultural issues. Essential reading for anyone concerned with worldwide issues in breastfeeding.

The Art of Breastfeeding, La Leche League International, August Robertson, Australia and London 1988. A basic guide to breastfeeding for women. Adapted for women in the U.K., Ireland and Australia from the American version.

Breastfeeding and Human Lactation, Jan Riordan and Kathleen Auerbach (Jones and Bartlett Publishers, Boston and London, 1993). Written for health workers, this book provides answers to some of the more obscure problems. Widely referenced.

Shared Parenthood: A Handbook for Fathers, Johanna Roeber (London, Melbourne, and Auckland: Century Paperbacks, 1987). A well-written, sensible, and caring book about pregnancy, birth, and infant care from the father's point of view. Good discussions of men's feelings about breastfeeding.

World of the Newborn, Martin Richards (New York: Harper & Row, 1980). This book will tell you about a newborn baby's amazing range of abilities and will provide a general understanding of babies.

Enabling Women to Breastfeed, Mary Renfrew and Mike Woolridge. The Stationary Office, London, 2000. This up-to-date text gives guidance for practice and detailed information about research studies.

Feeding Twins, Triplets and More, Margie Davis and Jane Denton. Multiple Births Foundation, London, 1999.

The authors have been involved in the production of videos about breastfeeding. These include:

Breastfeeding—coping with the first week
Breastfeeding—dealing with the problems, and
Breastfeeding—focus on attachment

These can all be obtained from Robert Copeland, Mark-It Television Associates, 7 Quarry Way, Stapleton, Bristol BS16 1UP. Tel 0117 939 1117/8.
http://www.Markittv.com (in the UK), or from Childbirth Graphics, PO Box 21207, Waco, TX 76702-1207 USA. Tel (800) 299 3366 (in North America).

An Explanation of Terms Used in This Book

Anesthesia. *See* General, Epidural or Regional, or Spinal anesthesia

Areola. The circular, dark area around the nipples.

Breast abscess. An infected area in the breast that is swollen and tender and filled with pus. *See page 119.*

Breast pump. A device that helps extract milk from the breast. It works by suction and can be powered by hand, by battery, or by electricity. *See pages 86-88.*

Breast shells. Pieces of curved plastic or glass that fit inside the bra. Also called *milk cups*. It is claimed that they pull out inverted nipples, though this has never been proven. Some types can be used to collect excess breast milk.

Burping. Bringing up gas or wind.

Candida. *See* Thrush.

Colostrum. The thick, yellow milk produced in the first few days of breastfeeding. It is high in protein and protects the baby from infection. *See page 70.*

Demand feeding. *See* Flexible feeding.

Engorgement. Painful swelling of the breasts. *See pages 116.*

Epidural anesthesia. Anesthesia given to help delivery via a tube into the back. It numbs from the waist to the thighs and does not put the woman to sleep. It can be used to assist a normal or a cesarean section delivery. *See page 31.*

Flat nipples. *See* Nonprotractile nipples.

Flexible feeding. Feeding a baby when the mother and child decide the time is right rather than by a set schedule. Some people call this *demand feeding*; we prefer to think of it as feeding that suits both the mother and baby (flexible) rather than feeding that is demanded by the baby. *See page 72.*

Foremilk. The milk that the baby takes during the first few minutes of feeding. It has a high volume (good for the baby's fluid intake) and has a low fat concentration. A baby needs a balance of both foremilk and hindmilk.

General anesthetic. Anesthetic that puts a woman into a special state of consciousness to help either a cesarean section delivery or with complications of vaginal birth, such as retained afterbirth. *See page 31.*

Hindmilk. The milk that a baby takes after the first few minutes of feeding. It is lower in volume (so the feeding slows down) and higher in calories or fat (good for the baby's growth and energy level). A baby needs a good intake of both hind-milk and foremilk. *See pages 70-72.*

Inverted nipples. A nipple that turns inward rather than projecting outward, resembling a small crater. One or both nipples may be inverted. *See pages 91-92.*

Jaundice. A condition, quite common in the first few days after birth, where the baby's skin and eyes become yellow. Because it occurs for a number of reasons, it is important to discover the particular cause for each baby. *See pages 136-138.*

Letdown reflex. The breasts' release of milk for the baby. Some women experience it as a tingling sensation. It is caused by the hormone oxytocin. *See page 68*

Lochia. The loss of blood a woman experiences after the birth of a baby that continues for the first few weeks. Breastfeeding speeds up the process, so the flow is heavier but stops sooner. *See page 68.*

Mastitis. Red, inflamed breasts. *See page 117-118.*

Milk ejection reflex. *See* Letdown reflex.

Nipple shields. Thin, plastic shapes that fit over the nipple to offer protection from pain when the baby feeds. They can reduce the milk supply and can cause other problems. They are helpful in the long term in only a few situations.

Nonprotractile nipples. Flat nipples that will not project outward. *See pages 91-92.*

Oxytocin. The hormone released when a baby feeds or when the mother thinks about feeding. It causes the milk to be released (the letdown reflex). It is also released when a woman makes love. Synthetic preparations of this hormone, used to induce or accelerate labor, are marketed at Pitocin or as Syntocinon. *See page 68.*

Prolactin. The hormone released when feeding a baby that causes the breasts to produce more milk. It plays an important part in the supply and demand mechanism. *See page 66.*

Regional anesthesia. This term is sometimes used to describe both epidural and spinal anesthesia. See the listings for these terms.

Spinal anesthesia. Anesthesia that numbs the lower part of the body but does not put the individual to sleep. It is administered via a needle in the back.

Thrush. An infection that occurs most commonly in the vagina or in a baby's mouth and digestive system. Also known as *candida* or *yeast infection.* It is caused by an overabundance of yeasts that are normally present in the body. Symptoms are a white discharge in the vagina or white flecks on a baby's tongue and cheeks. *See pages 123-124.*

Yeast infection. *See* Thrush.

BIBLIOGRAPHY

THE information in this book is based on extensive reading of research as well as on clinical experience. We have read and reviewed hundreds of books and articles; this listing contains some of the work that has been most helpful.

Ardran, G. M., F. H. Kemp, and J. Lind, "A Cineradiographic Study of Bottle Feeding." *British Journal of Radiology* 31 (1958): 11-12.

———— "A Cineradiographic Study of Breastfeeding." *British Journal of Radiology* 31 (1958): 156-162.

Auerbach, K. G., and L. M. Gartner. "Breastfeeding and Human Milk: Their Association with Jaundice in the Neonate." *Clinics in Perinatology* 14, no. 1 (1987): 89-107.

Coutsoudis, A., Pillay, K., Spooner, E. et al. "Influence of infant-feeding patterns on early mother-to-child transmission of HIV-1 in Durban, South Africa: a prospective cohort study.: *Lancet* 354 (1999) pp 471-473

European Collaborative Study. "Mother-to-Child Transmission of HIV Infection." *Lancet* 2, no. 8619 (1988): 1039-1042.

Foster, K., Lader, S., and Cheesbrough, S. *Infant Feeding 1995*. Office for National Statistics, The Stationary Office, London, 1997

Garza, C., R. J. Schanler, N. F. Butte, and K. J. Motil. "Special Properties of Human Milk." *Clinics in Perinatology* 14, no. 1 (1987): 11-32.

Gunther, M. *Infant Feeding*. London: Methuen, 1971.

Hall, B. "Changing Composition of Milk and Early Development of an Appetite Control." *Lancet* 1. no. 7910 (1975): 779-781.

Howie, P.W. Forsyth, J.S., Ogston, S.A., Clark, A., Florey, C. V. "Protective effect of breastfeeding." *British Medical Journal* 300 (1990): 11-16.

Hira, S.K., Mangrola, U.G., Murale, C., Chintu, C., Tembo, A., Brady, W.E., and Periue, P. L. "Apparent vertical transmission of human immunodeficiency virus type 1 by breastfeeding in Zambia." *The Journal of Pediatrics* 117 (1990): 421-424.

Hytten, F. "Clinical Studies in Lactation, II: Variations in the Major Constituents During a Feeding." *British Medical Journal* 1 (1954): 176-179.

Illingworth, R. S. and D. G. H. Stone. "Self-Demand Feeding in a Maternity Unit." *Lancet* 1, no. 14 (1952): 683-687.

Inch, S., and S. Garforth. "Establishing and Maintaining Lactation." In *Effective Care in Pregnancy and Childbirth*, ed. I. Chalmers, M. Enkin, and M. J. N. C. Kierse. Oxford: Oxford University Press, 1989.

Inch, S., and M. Renfrew. "Common Breastfeeding Problems." In *Effective Care in Pregnancy and Childbirth*, ed. I. Chalmers, M. Enkin, and M. J. N. C. Kierse. Oxford: Oxford University Press, 1989.

Italian Multicentre Study. "Epidemiology, Clinical Features, and Prognostic Factors of Paediatric HIV Infection." *Lancet* 2, no. 8619 (1988): 1043-1046.

Lepage, P., et al. "Postnatal Transmission of HIV from Mother to Child." [letter] *Lancet* 2, no. 8555 (1987): 400.

Lissauer, T. "Impact of AIDS on Neonatal Care." *Archives of Disease in Childhood* 64 (1989): 4-7.

Lucas, A. & Cole, T.J. "Breastmilk and Neonatal necrotising enterocolitis." *Lancet* 336 (1990): 15 19-1523

Martin, J. and A. White. *Infant Feeding: 1985 Office of Population Censuses and Surveys.* London: Her Majesty's Stationery Office, 1988.

McNeilly, A. S., I. C. Robinson, M. J. Houston, and P. W. Howie. "Release of Oxytocin and Prolactin in Response to Suckling." *British Medical Journal* 286 (1983): 257-259.

Meier, P. "Bottle and Breast Feeding Effects on Transcutaneous Oxygen Pressure and Temperature in Preterm Infants." *Nursing Research* 37 (1988): 36-41.

Minchin, M. *Breastfeeding Matters.* Melbourne, Australia: Alma Publications, 1998.

Nutrition Committee of the Canadian Paediatric Society and the Committee of Nutrition of the American Academy of Pediatrics. "Breast-feeding: A Commentary in Celebration of the International Year of the Child." *Pediatrics* 62 (1978): 591-601.

Royal College of Midwives. *Successful Breast-feeding: A Practical Guide for Midwives and Others Supporting Breastfeeding Mothers.* Churchill Livingstone, Edinburgh, 1993.

Renfrew, M. J., Woolridge, M. W., and Ross McGill, H. *Enabling women to breastfeed: a review of practices which support or hinder breastfeeding, with evidence-based guidance for practice.* The Stationary Office, London, 2000.

Saliriya, E. M., P. M. Easton, and J. I. Cater. "Duration of Breast-Feeding After Early Initiation and Frequent Feeding." *Lancet* 2, no. 8100 (1978): 1141-1143.

Thapa, S., R. V. Short, and M. Potts. "Breast-feeding, Birth Spacing and Their Effects on Child Survival." *Nature* 335 (1988): 679-682.

Thomsen, A. C., et al. "Course and Treatment of Milk Stasis, Non-Infectious Inflammation of the Breast and Infectious Mastitis in Nursing Women." *American Journal of Obstetrics and Gynecology* 149, no. 5 (1984): 492-495.

Uvnas-Moberg, K. "The Gastrointestinal Tract in Growth and Reproduction." *Scientific American*, July 1989, 78-83.

Verronen, P. "Breastfeeding: Reasons for Giving Up and Transient Lactational Crises." *Acta Pediatrica Scandinavia* 71 (1982): 447-450.

Widstrom, A. M., et al. "Gastric Suction in Healthy Newborn Infants." *Acta Pediatrica Scandinavica* 76 (1987): 556-572.

Wilson, A. C., Forsyth, J. S., Greene, S. S., et al. "Relation of diet to childhood health: seven year follow-up of cohort of children in Dundee infant feeding study." *British Medical Journal* 316 (1988): 21-25.

Woolridge, M. W. "The Anatomy of Infant Sucking, and the Aetiology of Sore Nipples." *Midwifery*, 2 (1986): 164-176.

Woolridge, M. W. and C. Fisher. "Colic, Overfeeding, and Symptoms of Lactose Malabsorption in the Breast-Fed Baby: A Possible Artifact of Feed Management?" *Lancet* 2, no. 8607 (1988): 382-384.

World Health Organisation. A Review of HIV transmission through breastfeeding WHO, Geneva, 1998.

Index of Commonly Asked Questions

Index

More Books on women's health and family issues . . .

Special Delivery by Rahima Baldwin

Midwife, childbirth educator, and internationally-known speaker Rahima Baldwin presents a guide to structuring the birth experience you want for yourself and your baby. Chapters cover choosing hospital or home birth, prenatal care, handling labor, dealing with complications, and more.

Pregnant Feelings by Rahima Baldwin & Terra Palmarini Richardson

This workbook for pregnant women and their partners helps them to recognize and work with the emotions and energies surrounding pregnancy and birth. Practical exercises lead to a sense of self-confidence and power in new and not-so-new parents.

Women Giving Birth by Saskiavan Rees, Beatris Smulders, & Astrid Limburg

Profusely illustrated with color photographs, this important new book on natural childbirth covers the latest research into drug-free labor, vertical delivery (an ancient but little-known birthing technique), and water births.

Hearts & Hands by Elizabeth Davis

This comprehensive and classic "midwife's guide" to pregnancy and birth demystifies modern obstetrics and provides sound guidelines for alternative care. Illustrated with line drawings and more than 60 photographs by Suzanne Arms.

After the Baby's Birth . . . A Woman's Way to Wellness by Robin Lim

This complete guide to postpartum care for mother and baby focuses on natural and wholesome practices. Illustrated throughout, this warm, sensitive text has advice on parental nurturing, breast-feeding, nutrition, pelvic health, early education, the role of the father, and the all-importance of love.

You Are Your Child's First Teacher by Rahima Baldwin

An exciting new vision of parenting in which parents have an active educational role from the moment of birth. Drawing on child development research, Baldwin details how to nurture your child's mind, body, emotions, and imagination.

Available from your local bookstore, or order directly from the publisher.

Celestial Arts, P.O. Box 7123, Berkeley, CA 94707

For VISA, Mastercard, or American Express orders call (800) 841-book.